Minding Your
Memory

Minding Your Memory

What You Can Do Now to Prevent Dementia and Stay Sharp for Life

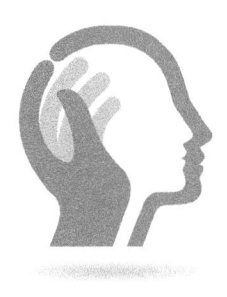

Written by Members of the
Sharp Again Medical Advisory Board

EDITED BY
Lisa Feiner and Steve Ledvina

Sharp Again
White Plains, NY

Minding Your Memory: What You Can Do Now to Prevent Dementia and Stay Sharp for Life
©2025, Sharp Again Naturally LLC DBA Sharp Again

All rights reserved. This book or any portion thereof may not be reproduced or used in any manner whatsoever without the express written permission of the publisher except for the use of brief quotations in a book review.

For information about permission to reproduce selections from this book, contact info@sharpagain.org. Visit sharpagain.org to learn more.

First printing: 2025

This book was created with help from Editwright.
Visit editwright.com for more information.

Developmental editing by Andrew Doty
Copyediting by Allison Janicki
Book design and cover design by Peggy Nehmen, n-kcreative.com
Proofreading by Karen L. Tucker
Published by Sharp Again

Typeset in Acumin Pro, National and Sabon

ISBN Print: 979-8-9926978-0-3
ISBN Ebook: 979-8-9926978-2-7
Library of Congress Control Number: 2025911834

*This book is dedicated to everyone
who has lost a loved one to Alzheimer's disease
and other dementias.*

*With the information in this book, we hope
that throughout your life
you will retain your personhood,
your relationships with family and friends,
and engagement with the passions
and pursuits you truly love.*

Contents

Contributors and Editors 1
Foreword 3
Introduction 7

Part One: Lifestyle Factors 17
1. Nutrition and Supplements 21
2. Physical Activity 39
3. Mental Stimulation 51
4. Social Interaction 55
5. Sleep and Breathing 59
6. Prolonged Stress 75

Part Two: The Deeper Dive 89
7. Hormones 91
8. Toxins 105
9. Heavy Metal Toxicity 129
10. Inflammation and Infections 147
11. Prescription Medication 171
12. Physical and Emotional Trauma 181

Part Three: Don't Wait — Act Today! 201
13. Finding Qualified Healthcare Professionals 203
14. Additional Reading 207

Acknowledgments 211
Glossary 213
Endnotes 225

Contributors and Editors

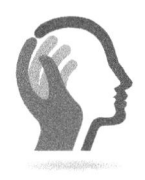

CONTRIBUTORS
Richard Carlton, MD
Michael Gelb, DDS
Howard Hindin, DDS
Robert Kachko, ND LAc
Gary Klingsberg, DO
Cornelia Lenherr, MD
David Lerner, DDS
Shanhong Lu, MD
Penelope McDonnell, ND
Ilene Naomi Rusk, PhD
Susanne Saltzman, MD
Allan Warshowsky, MD

EDITORS
Lisa Feiner, MBA, MEd, NBC-HWC
Steve Ledvina, NBC-HWC

ASSOCIATE EDITOR
Barbara Goldenberg, MBA

Foreword

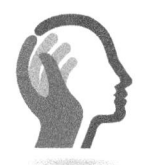

WE ARE LIVING AT A PIVOTAL moment in the history of brain health — an inflection point where, for the first time, the conversation around memory loss is shifting from helplessness to hope, from inevitability to empowerment. *Minding Your Memory*, edited by Lisa Feiner and Steve Ledvina, stands as a beacon of empowerment in this transformation. This book is a rallying call for those of us who refuse to wait passively for cognitive decline to strike and instead choose to actively safeguard their mental vitality.

For far too long, the prevailing narrative around Alzheimer's disease and other forms of dementia has been one of despair — focused on diagnosis, decline, and, eventually, dependence. While pharmaceutical interventions have been pursued with great energy, the results have fallen far short of what we had hoped. Despite billions of dollars invested in research, there remains no effective drug that can meaningfully reverse the trajectory of Alzheimer's disease. And yet, *Minding Your Memory* reminds us that this is not the whole story.

The authors assembled by Feiner and Ledvina have masterfully explored the growing body of scientific evidence showing that we can, in fact, take meaningful steps — starting today — to reduce our risk of dementia. This book is grounded in the recognition that our brain health is not sealed by fate or genetics alone. Rather, it is shaped daily by our lifestyle choices, by our environments, and by our willingness to engage with a systems-based, root-cause approach to wellness.

What makes this book so timely and powerful is that it doesn't simply tell us what's wrong; it illuminates what's possible. It unpacks a multitude of modifiable factors — ranging from nutrition, sleep, and exercise to toxin exposure, stress, trauma, and even the overlooked contributions of oral health and gut integrity — that contribute to memory decline. Each of these is an invitation: an opening to take back agency in a space that once seemed hopelessly deterministic.

The evidence is compelling. We now understand that memory loss is not an inevitable part of aging but often the downstream result of systemic imbalances — metabolic dysfunction, chronic inflammation, and immune dysregulation, to name a few. Crucially, *Minding Your Memory* not only presents these insights with clarity and scientific rigor, but it also provides the tools to act on them. Whether you're a layperson concerned about your cognitive future, a family member supporting a loved one, or a clinician seeking to integrate cutting-edge prevention strategies, this book meets you where you are.

Feiner and Ledvina have long been leaders in the field of cognitive resilience. Their deep personal connections to the topic, combined with their professional expertise as board-certified health coaches, make this work not only evidence-based, but also deeply human. Their work through Sharp Again offers a model of what patient-centered, preventive care can look like in the 21st century.

This book doesn't offer one magic bullet — because there isn't one. What it offers is something far more powerful: a comprehensive, integrative framework for protecting the most precious asset we have — our minds. It champions a future in which cognitive decline is no longer viewed as a sentence but as a solvable challenge. The message here is loud and clear: Cognitive decline is, to a significant extent, preventable.

Let this book serve as your guide, your reference, and your inspiration. It is a beacon for a new era in brain health, where knowledge is power, action is medicine, and hope is entirely justified.

—David Perlmutter, MD
Board-certified neurologist
Author of #1 *New York Times* bestsellers *Grain Brain* and *Drop Acid*

Introduction

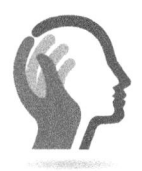

THIS BOOK IS ABOUT HOPE. For the first time, it's possible to take action to maintain our brain health, prevent and delay cognitive decline and dementia, and remain mentally sharp throughout our lives.

Many of the underlying causes of Alzheimer's disease (AD) and other dementias have just recently been identified and are becoming better understood. Research studies over the past 15 years show that lifestyle and daily habits, exposure to environmental toxins, history of stress and trauma, and many other factors have a complex interplay with our physiology and can be modified to decrease our risk of AD. We have come to understand that the body and brain are a "system of systems," and therefore, there are ways to influence various aspects of our bodies and brains to improve the brain's aging process.

Alzheimer's disease and related dementias are terms that are often used interchangeably, but they are not the same. Dementia is a broad category of symptoms and diseases that can have many etiologies, including Lewy body dementia, frontotemporal dementia, vascular dementia, Parkinson's-related dementia, and Alzheimer's disease. These are all neurodegenerative diseases which result in progressive neuropsychological dysfunction that may manifest as memory issues, difficulty with using the correct words, poor judgment and decision-making (executive function), spatial issues, hallucinations, and/or other neurocognitive changes.

Alzheimer's pathology is the most common type of dementia and is estimated to be 60 to 70 percent of all cases. The pathology of AD is characterized by several physiological changes, most notably the buildup of beta amyloid outside of neurons and the aggregation of phosphorylated tau inside cells in certain brain regions; it is often accompanied by inflammation and tiny vascular changes in the brain as well. *The Lancet* estimates that on a global basis, the number of people with dementia will increase from 57.4 million cases in 2019 to 152.8 million cases in 2050,[1] which underscores the need to understand the underlying causes of memory loss, associated treatment protocols, and prevention strategies.

When Sharp Again began gathering information in 2012 about causes of memory loss, few people were aware that patients diagnosed with AD could be — and had been — treated and their memory loss reversed. Because this was such a new idea, the founders of the organization decided to aggregate research studies, clinical reports, periodicals, and other resource materials to help identify the likely causes of memory loss, and we continue to monitor new research as it becomes available. For this reason, *Minding Your Memory* includes over 500 citations, enabling the medical community and the public to see how the understanding of memory loss has progressed and to dig more deeply into the science if they choose. We believe this is a unique endeavor and is necessary to change the beliefs, perspective, and clinical treatment around Alzheimer's and other dementias.

As Sharp Again began sharing this research with the public, more factors that potentially impact cognition were brought to our attention, often by those who attended our presentations. The causal nature of these risk factors was fully researched as well. In partnership with the medical and dental professionals on our Medical Advisory Board, Sharp Again established a list of causes of memory loss. *Minding Your Memory* discusses each of the following risk factors in depth:

- Nutritional imbalances and deficiencies
- Inadequate physical activity
- Insufficient mental stimulation
- Social isolation
- Sleep and breathing problems
- Prolonged stress
- Hormonal imbalances
- Toxins in food, water, air, and work/home environment
- Mercury and other heavy metal toxicity
- Inflammation from low-level infections
- Effects of prescription medications
- Physical and emotional trauma

Other risk factors are correlated with memory loss, and this list has been growing substantially. Sharp Again has not yet categorized them as confirmed causes per se, as more research is needed. However, it has become clear that many of these risk factors, when left untreated, often lead to memory loss. These include cardiovascular disease, obesity, hearing loss, vision loss (glaucoma), depression, and diabetes.

In addition, smoking and heavy alcohol use have long been associated with myriad health risks. Research studies have shown that continued smoking is also strongly associated with dementia,[2,3] with the World Health Organization (WHO) estimating that 14 percent of dementia cases worldwide may be caused by smoking.[4] Some studies show that consuming alcohol above the 21-drink weekly threshold leads to a higher likelihood of cognitive decline and hippocampal atrophy.[5]

The 2020 *Lancet* report on Dementia Prevention, Intervention, and Care discusses 12 risk factors and suggests that modifying them "might prevent or delay up to 40% of dementias."[6] As additional research is undertaken, the causal nature of these conditions will become more evident, and Sharp Again will make this new information available.

Genes, Epigenetics, and Alzheimer's Disease

Many genes impact brain function, most particularly the apolipoprotein E (ApoE) gene. Each person receives one copy of this gene from their mother and one copy from their father, each one with a numeric allele of E2, E3, or E4 at the end. These are known as gene variants. Researchers have found that having one or two copies of the ApoE4 genetic variant increases the risk of developing AD. The ApoE4 variant has also been associated with elevated cholesterol levels and increased risk of cardiovascular disease. Only 2 to 3 percent of people are homozygous for ApoE4, meaning they have two copies. People who inherit two copies of the ApoE4 gene, called ApoE4 homozygotes, have a 60 percent chance of developing AD by age 85. However, people who have two copies of this variant comprise only 15 percent of Alzheimer's cases. So it is clear that genetics play a role but will not necessarily determine that someone will develop Alzheimer's. There is a complex interplay between genes and environmental factors that determines this outcome.

Epigenetics is the relationship between our genes and how they change in reaction to our environment and how we live. The evidence presented in this book illustrates numerous root causes of Alzheimer's and dementia above and beyond our genetic risk. Genes are turned on or off based on many factors, including lifestyle, exposure to toxins, stress and trauma, and the condition of our immune system. Developing and incorporating healthy, science-supported lifestyle habits into one's daily routine is clearly a beneficial strategy for minimizing risk for Alzheimer's as well as other diseases.

Today, people who are homozygous for ApoE4 are maintaining their cognition throughout their lives by following a multi-therapeutic approach to brain health. Knowing one's ApoE status may empower those carrying the ApoE4 genetic variant to start taking active steps in their 30s and 40s to keep their brains and bodies functioning at optimal levels. As with any chronic health condition, the earlier one starts, the greater the likelihood that Alzheimer's can be delayed or prevented altogether.

Advances in Testing

New blood tests for Alzheimer's disease have made significant strides, offering a less invasive, cost-effective method for detecting early signs of the condition. Recent tests measure specific biomarkers, particularly phosphorylated tau proteins (like p-tau217 and p-tau181), which can indicate Alzheimer's pathology up to 10 years before symptoms emerge. These tests show great promise and accuracy in clinical and research settings, and some are already commercially available. Ongoing validation and clinical approval processes will continue to broaden their widespread adoption.

How This Book Came to Be

An early goal of Sharp Again was to aggregate and share all of the modifiable risk factors for cognitive decline and AD and realize its mission to educate people by documenting the scientific research that supported the causes of, and treatments for, cognitive decline. Many clinicians in the traditional medical community are skeptical of the multi-therapeutic approach because it is difficult to carry out a double-blind, placebo-controlled trial on such an array of variables. This type of approach does not allow for testing one drug or intervention at a time, but recently, several studies have been carried out using this multimodal approach[7, 8] with positive outcomes for patients. The research contained herein supports the numerous root contributors to the development of AD, and using this multi-therapeutic treatment approach has shown cognition to improve in up to 84 percent of cases.[9] Members of the Sharp Again Board and its Medical Advisory Board, as well as our greater community, spent countless hours reviewing the research, and we will continue to periodically revise the material both online and in future editions of this book as new research becomes available.

Minding Your Memory brings together not only information on the underlying causes of memory loss but also symptoms and considerations for testing and treatment. Some chapters present questions for both patients and practitioners to consider on the road to healing. This material is based on both our advisory board doctors' clinical experience as well as our coaches' experience with individual clients and those in the Sharp Again group coaching program. Taking charge of our health and well-being usually starts with small steps that together, over time, create true change and ultimately better health.

Who This Book Is For

MOST SHARP AGAIN PUBLICATIONS ARE DESIGNED for the layperson so that the information on the causes and treatment of memory loss are within the grasp of every individual and their family members. Our *Road Map to a Sharper Mind* is a 20-page guide that provides basic information and suggestions about what steps to take if one wants to begin learning about the underlying causes of memory loss or is experiencing memory lapses.[10] *Minding Your Memory* is an amplification of that guide, containing expanded discussions on symptoms, varied approaches for addressing the causes, and considerations when seeking treatment. Finding Qualified Healthcare Professionals explains how readers can find a doctor in their area, and an Additional Reading list provides books that go into greater detail on some topics than we do here.

This book is also to be used as a companion guide and reference for the Sharp Again group coaching programs. The programs are designed for people who are worried about their cognition because they have started to notice memory issues, have a family history of Alzheimer's, or want to become educated about brain health. By addressing many of the modifiable lifestyle factors, participants can start to improve their memory and overall health and well-being.

Minding Your Memory is also for medical professionals and others who are motivated to understand the science supporting the causal relationships for dementia and who wish to explore the research in depth. Medical terminology is used, and references to research studies and other relevant citations are provided. Healthcare practitioners who want to better understand how cognition is impacted by these factors and the relevant treatment options will also find the book helpful. A glossary and resources for additional reading are provided at the end of the book.

As You Read This Book

It is important to bear in mind that each person is unique in their biology, lifestyle, history, and personality. Although our genetics may resemble those of family members, we each have our individual genetic makeup, and the ways in which those genes are expressed are individual as well. Over our lifetime, we develop particular habits, such as the foods we eat, the quantity and quality of our sleep, whether we exercise and what types of movement we enjoy, and so on. We may have been exposed to traumatic experiences and other external factors such as toxins, viruses, and diseases that shape our biology and our mental state. We are able to benefit from the research that shows how effective lifestyle changes and other interventions can be in improving our overall health and well-being.

This book is divided into two sections: Lifestyle Factors and The Deeper Dive. Lifestyle factors can often be addressed by individuals on their own, with family support, or by working with a health coach. The causes of memory loss discussed in The Deeper Dive require testing and treatment by qualified medical professionals and are often the product of exposures in the environment or life experiences. Testing is available to help diagnose these causes and provide direction for treatment. We encourage everyone to work with a primary care physician or integrative practitioner, or to seek the advice of other qualified healthcare clinicians, including someone who can perform a neuropsychological evaluation and other appropriate testing.

A health coach, especially one trained in the prevention and treatment of cognitive decline, can also be a valuable member of your team. Health coaches can be the conduit between doctor and patient, helping patients to implement a physician's recommendations and put them into action and keeping clients motivated and on track.

This book is by no means an exhaustive analysis of the causes of memory loss and is intended to be an ongoing and evolving discussion that reflects the new scientific studies and discoveries that are made every day. We hope you find it valuable and welcome your comments at info@sharpagain.org.

About Sharp Again

Founded in 2012 as a not-for-profit organization, the original mission of Sharp Again was to educate individuals, their families, and caregivers, as well as the medical and dental professionals supporting them, about causes of memory loss and dementia, with the hope of reducing the number of new cases of Alzheimer's disease. In the past several years, the focus has shifted toward prevention and early intervention because, in most cases, it is much easier to prevent memory loss than it is to treat it. It has also become clear that, while education about the causes of memory loss is critically important, hearing or seeing the information is not enough. The missing link is taking the information and putting it into action by integrating new habits and practices into daily life.

The editors of the book, Lisa Feiner and Steve Ledvina, are nationally board-certified health coaches with personal and professional experience in the field of dementia care and prevention. Lisa, a cofounder of Sharp Again, has dedicated over 25 years to working with elders, both as a volunteer and board member at a skilled nursing and rehabilitation facility. Her journey into dementia care began when she learned about individuals diagnosed with Alzheimer's disease who had regained cognition after being treated for the underlying causes of their condition. This discovery deeply resonated with her, as it highlighted the potential for treating dementia through a better understanding of its root causes, similar to other diseases.

Steve's involvement in dementia care is rooted in personal experience, having lost three grandparents to dementia. This personal connection led him to shift his career gradually, focusing on helping individuals prevent and manage the disease. Both Lisa and Steve have undergone extensive training to work with individuals who have dementia in their families or are experiencing early signs of cognitive decline, offering guidance and support in managing or preventing the progression of memory-related conditions.

Today, the mission of Sharp Again is to educate the public and the medical community about causes of memory loss and empower every individual to optimize their cognitive health and overall well-being. We achieve this through education and coaching programs that help people identify action steps for improvement and that offer support in the areas of nutrition, sleep, exercise, stress, social relationships, and mental engagement. Additional contributing factors such as exposure to toxins and heavy metals, hormone imbalances, inflammation due to infections, and trauma require treatment and are best addressed with appropriate medical professionals.

Sharp Again is a valuable resource for everyone who wants to start on the road to cognitive and overall health. Our primary audience is the "worried well" — people who have a family history of dementia or who are concerned about their own memory. We also collaborate with healthcare practitioners who want to learn more about the causes of memory loss and how they can be addressed. Our Foundational Coaching Program and Maintain Your Brain group participants actively work with health coaches in a group setting to learn ways to enhance cognition and keep their minds sharp. Through this effort, Sharp Again is part of a growing and urgent effort to stem the rise of Alzheimer's and other dementias worldwide.

Ten years ago, no one thought memory loss was treatable, much less reversible; a multi-therapeutic approach was outside the mainstream of traditional medicine. Today, with the wealth of research and new understanding of the brain's capabilities, Sharp Again is in lockstep with forward-thinking practitioners who have seen the power of lifestyle and environmental interventions, brain training, and treatment of chronic infections, hormonal imbalances, and physical and emotional trauma to measurably improve a person's cognitive function. We envision a world where dementia can be prevented, treated, and reversed — and where everyone has access to the knowledge, tools, and care needed to preserve their cognition throughout their lives.

PART ONE
LIFESTYLE FACTORS

THERE HAS BEEN NO SHORTAGE of advice from every corner of the healthcare community about the importance of adopting a healthy lifestyle, including exercising regularly, getting regular sleep, managing stress, staying socially connected, and keeping mentally engaged. This advice is increasingly supported by substantial research data. Multiple studies have found that these factors are among the critical determinants of brain and overall health and — both individually and in combination — can keep the body healthy and prevent dementia.

The risk factors associated with lifestyle practices are intricately woven into our daily lives and are primarily within our control. For many people, interventions in these lifestyle factors, along with improved nutrition, have helped restore mental function considerably, so these measures can be thought of as both potential causes of dementia and a powerful preventive solution to ward off cognitive decline.

One of the most significant studies in this area is the Finnish Geriatric Intervention Study to Prevent Cognitive Impairment and Disability (FINGER),[11] the first randomized controlled trial showing that it is possible to prevent cognitive decline using a multidomain lifestyle intervention among older individuals who are at risk for dementia.

The study showed that the combination of nutritional guidance, physical exercise, cognitive training, social activities, and management of vascular and metabolic risk factors improved cognition in the treatment group, even among those with a genetic predisposition for dementia. After two years, participants experienced an approximately 25 percent improvement in cognition.[12] The study is ongoing and has expanded worldwide. The results confirm that dementia often has roots in our basic lifestyle practices, and addressing these practices can help prevent or delay the onset of cognitive decline.

Studies have also shown that mental, physical, and social leisure activities have a protective effect against dementia.[13] Persistent engagement in effortful mental activities may even promote changes in the brain that can help to delay symptoms of underlying dementia pathology.[14] Physical activity increases cerebral oxygenation, leading to improved neurotransmitter metabolism. It also reduces the risk of health conditions that are risk factors for dementia such as hypertension, diabetes, and cardiovascular disease.[15, 16] Predominantly social leisure activities may have beneficial effects on the immune system,[17] which in turn could influence inflammatory processes in the brain which are strongly associated with dementia. Each of these lifestyle factors will be addressed separately to better illustrate the research supporting their link to cognitive health.

Combining Lifestyle Factors for a Healthier Brain

Research also shows that combining two or more lifestyle factors can have a synergistic effect on brain health. A study in Germany compared the effects of an 18-month specially designed dance program that required participants to constantly learn new choreographies against a traditional health fitness training program of mainly repetitive exercises. Participants were learning new steps, socializing with others, and getting exercise through dance. At the end of the study, participants in both groups showed increases in the volume of the hippocampus region of the brain — a region critical for memory consolidation. However, the dance group showed greater increases in volume as well as improved balance.[18] Another study of Japanese men and women with an average age of 76 who exercised with others compared to those who exercised alone had a lower risk of dementia as well.[19]

Studies have also looked at the combination of cognitive training and motor training (known as dual-task training) and found that each has benefits, but together they have a greater impact on cognition.[20] In another study, resistance training and cognitive training together were shown to increase brain-derived neurotrophic factor (BDNF) and enhance cognition.[21] People who engage in both types of activities typically have higher functionality and a better quality of life as well.

Nutrition, exercise, sleep, mental stimulation, social interaction, and managing stress are crucial for a healthy brain, no matter what our age. When we are young, these components of our lives may seem to come naturally, and combining these activities can also be fun and challenging. As we age, however, many people start to have deficits in one or more areas and have to work harder at keeping their lives in balance. Each of these lifestyle factors is examined in detail in this section.

1

Nutrition and Supplements

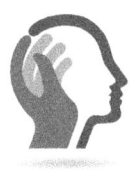

OVER A LIFETIME, NUTRITION HAS A profound effect on the health of the body and the brain. Many studies show the Mediterranean diet or other similar diets rich in plant-based foods provide support for brain function. Individuals would be wise to consult a physician before making significant changes to diet and supplementation.

Research has also shown that certain nutrition-based lifestyle factors, including eating patterns (how we eat, when we eat, etc.) and consumption of specific foods and their micronutrients support cognitive well-being into old age. It is important to remember that everyone has a unique body, health history, and family history; therefore, there is no universal "ideal" diet.

In the past several decades, as our food has become more processed and industrialized, hormones, antibiotics, and genetically modified organisms (GMOs) have been used to keep livestock and plants from being infected (or infested) with a range of diseases. While this may have helped increase our food supply, it has also caused health problems for those consuming the food — after all, we are not only "what we eat" but also "what we eat eats."

Every year, new diets become popular, but where brain health is concerned, the research has been consistent. A recommended dietary protocol for brain health comprises:

- A nutritional foundation built on the Mediterranean-DASH Intervention for Neurodegenerative Delay (MIND) diet
- Sufficient hydration
- Use of beneficial herbs and spices
- Calorie monitoring and possible restriction
- Time-restricted feeding and intermittent fasting
- Ketogenic diet for those with insulin resistance
- Supplementation as needed
- Food sensitivity diagnosis and treatment

There are common mechanisms by which certain recommendations promote brain health and reduce Alzheimer's risk. These recommendations, sourced from specific research studies, include reducing inflammation, correcting insulin resistance, reducing oxidative stress, releasing molecules that help nerve cells regenerate, releasing trophic factors, and optimizing brain nutrition.[22, 23] These factors are interrelated; therefore, these recommendations may improve brain health through multiple mechanisms at once.

Build a Nutritional Foundation on the MIND Diet

The Mediterranean-DASH Intervention for Neurodegenerative Delay (MIND) diet protects the brain from cognitive decline and reduces Alzheimer's risk. In a 2014 study showing that the MIND diet reduced cognitive decline, the authors described the dietary regimen as a hybrid of the heart-healthy DASH (Dietary Approaches to Stop Hypertension) diet and the health-promoting Mediterranean diet with the addition of specific brain-healthy foods.[24] Although the DASH diet was originally developed to address high blood pressure, both regimens follow similar dietary guidelines (see the table on p. 24), with the exception of salt, which is more restricted in the DASH diet. In a 4.5-year study of 923 seniors, the same authors found the MIND diet lowered Alzheimer's risk by 35 percent for those with moderate adherence to the diet and

53 percent with high adherence when compared with participants with low adherence.[25] While further research would strengthen the case, a 2019 review of 56 studies concluded that following the MIND diet was associated with decreased cognitive decline and Alzheimer's disease risk.[26] In a 2023 study, women who followed a DASH diet also reported experiencing less cognitive decline later in life.[27]

Put the MIND Diet Into Practice

This section presents the general instructions for the MIND diet, followed by further recommendations by the Sharp Again Medical Advisory Board to make the diet even more supportive of brain health. Working with their healthcare providers, individuals can determine their optimal diets.

The MIND diet is a whole-food, plant-based diet, primarily consisting of vegetables, berries, whole grains, legumes, and nuts. The consumption of grains should be in moderation and in the form of whole grains to optimize nutritional value and reduce the potential to raise blood sugar. Adding healthy fats and various herbs and spices increases flavor and may reduce the need for salt. Red meat is limited, but fish and poultry may be eaten in moderation. Dairy products should be consumed in smaller amounts. For dessert, fresh fruit such as berries is recommended. The specific guidelines are shown in the following table, with foods to include at the top and foods to curtail at the bottom. All amounts listed are serving sizes that vary based on the particular food.

MIND Diet	
Foods to Add	**How Often**
Whole grains (1/2 cup)	≥ 3 per day
Green leafy vegetables (2 cups per serving)	≥ 6 per week
Other vegetables (1 cup)	≥ 1 per day
Berries (1 cup)	≥ 2 per week
Fish (3-5 oz.)	≥ 1 per week
Poultry (3-5 oz.)	≥ 2 per week
Beans (1/2 cup dry or 1 cup cooked)	> 3 per week
Nuts (1 oz.)	≥ 5 per week
Extra virgin olive oil	Use as primary oil
Foods to Limit	**How Often**
Red meats and meat products (3-5 oz.)	< 4 per week
Fast/fried food (3-5 oz. or comparable take-out serving)	< 1 per week
Butter, margarine (1 tbsp.)	< 1 per day
Cheese (2 oz.)	< 1 per week
Pastries, sweets (1 piece)	< 5 per week
Alcohol/wine (5 oz.)	1 per day

Include Brain-Healthy Foods Every Day

Berries

Fresh and frozen blueberries, raspberries, strawberries, and blackberries have anti-inflammatory and antioxidant (reduction of oxidative stress) properties and are relatively low in sugar. Other fruits, such as grapes, bananas, pineapples, and dried fruits may raise blood sugar quickly, so monitor your intake.[28, 29, 30]

Caffeine

Studies show that regular coffee and caffeine consumption promotes brain health and reduces the risk of Alzheimer's.[31, 32] However, for many people, it is advisable to limit or monitor caffeine intake after lunch so that sleep is not disrupted. Increasing awareness about whether ingesting caffeine causes anxiety, agitation, or problems falling asleep will determine how or if someone is adversely affected.

Coconut Oil
Medium-chain triglycerides (MCTs) are a type of saturated fat found in coconut oil that may be beneficial for the brain.[33] These fats convert into "ketone bodies" in the liver. While the body typically uses glucose for energy, in those individuals with insulin resistance, ketones are an alternative energy source for the body and the brain. Our bodies naturally produce ketones when we are in a fasting state; using coconut or MCT oil can be a way to jump-start the metabolic transition into ketosis, where the body is burning fat for energy instead of glucose. If using coconut oil for this purpose, it is important to select oils that do not contain hydrogenated fats (trans fats). Because coconut oil can cause loose stools, it is recommended that individuals start with just one teaspoon of extra virgin coconut oil per day and gradually work up to two tablespoons per day. There are differing views on the benefits of coconut oil and the appropriate dosages in the scientific and medical communities, so consulting one's physician is essential when considering adding it regularly to a diet.[34, 35]

Healthy Fats (Unsaturated)
Unsaturated fats promote brain health and include:
- **Monounsaturated Fats:** Almonds, avocados, olive oil, sesame seeds. These fats can help reduce the risk of heart disease and improve cholesterol, insulin, and blood sugar levels. Managing heart disease has been independently shown to reduce Alzheimer's risk.[36]
- **Polyunsaturated Fats:** Cold-water fish, pumpkin seeds, flaxseed, walnuts, oils. The polyunsaturated fats most associated with brain health and Alzheimer's prevention are Omega-3 fatty acids and two subtypes in particular, eicosapentaenoic acid (EPA) and docosahexaenoic acid (DHA), discussed in the Supplements section later

in this chapter. Unfortunately, many food labels do not show these subcategories of polyunsaturated fats, so being able to identify the foods that are good sources for them is valuable.

Herbs and Spices

Not only do herbs and spices provide flavor and variety to our meals, they also possess a host of advantageous qualities on their own, including antifungal, antiviral, antimicrobial, and anti-inflammatory properties, as well as containing polyphenols that help to prevent cellular damage.[37, 38] Turmeric and its active ingredient, curcumin, have been shown in studies to reduce inflammation, one of the leading causes of neurodegenerative diseases.[39] It is typically best combined with black pepper to increase bioavailability.

Saffron, a spice sold in powder form or in strands, has been shown in a small study to have positive effects for Alzheimer's patients.[40]

Herbs such as ashwagandha and bacopa monnieri also have a positive impact on the brain. A 2017 study of 50 participants over eight weeks concluded that "ashwagandha may be effective in enhancing both immediate and general memory in people with MCI (Mild Cognitive Impairment), as well as improving executive function, attention, and information processing speed."[41] Multiple studies have highlighted bacopa's ability to boost memory, cognitive skills, and multitasking.[42]

Hydration

Consuming clean, filtered water can help clear toxins, promote cellular health, reduce diabetes risk,[43] and contribute to overall health. Although the recommended amount of water to consume daily is highly individualized, a good rule of thumb is to drink the number of ounces per day equal to your body weight in pounds, divided by two (example: a 150-pound individual should drink 75 ounces of water per day). It is best to eliminate consumption of beverages high in sugar, such as fruit juices and sodas. Finally, it is important to note that any fluids that dehydrate the body, such as caffeinated coffee, teas, sodas, and alcohol, require additional water intake to compensate.

Olive Oil
As noted earlier, olive oil is rich in healthy monounsaturated fats. It also contains polyphenols, which have antioxidant and anti-inflammatory properties. Studies suggest that the cognitive protective effects in both the MIND and Mediterranean diets derive in part from the polyphenols in olive oil.[44, 45] Extra virgin olive oil (EVOO) has the most health-promoting properties due to its higher levels of antioxidants and is the least processed of all olive oils.

Prebiotics and Probiotics
Prebiotics and probiotics are important for the health of the gut microbiome. Prebiotics feed our good gut bacteria and consist of plant fibers that are found in a large range of foods such as Jerusalem artichokes; oats, barley, and other cereal grains; garlic, onion, and leeks; dandelion greens; chicory root; asparagus; bananas and apples; jicama, burdock, and konjac root; and seaweed and flaxseeds. Prebiotics not only help bowel function but also improve communication between the gut and the brain by producing neurotransmitters. Prebiotics also play a role in hormone development and enhance the body's immune function and anti-inflammatory response.[46]

Probiotic foods contain microorganisms that have a positive effect on digestion, mood, immunity, and heart health. Examples of probiotic foods are yogurt and kefir and fermented foods such as sauerkraut, kimchi, tempeh, miso, kombucha, and pickles. Probiotics can also be taken in supplement form.

Keeping the gut-brain axis healthy is important for a number of reasons. What happens in the gut also affects the brain and vice versa. This is primarily due to the vagus nerve that carries signals between your brain, heart, and digestive system. Research has shown that probiotics can have a positive effect on mood and cognition and may lower anxiety.[47, 48] In addition, research studies have shown that probiotic supplementation improved cognition in people with cognitive impairment and Alzheimer's.[49]

Wild-Caught Fatty Fish
Consuming baked or broiled fish such as wild salmon, lake trout, sardines, and mackerel at least twice per week is highly recommended.[50, 51] The cognitive benefits of fish may derive from more than just healthy fats, such as contributing to larger gray matter volume.[52] SMASH fish (salmon, mackerel, anchovies, sardines, and herring) are also recommended due to their low average mercury content.

Foods to Monitor, Minimize, or Eliminate

Alcohol
Light to moderate drinking has been associated with decreased risk for dementia and cognitive impairment,[53] with the recommended daily intake of one drink for women and one to two drinks for men. This finding was only relevant for those without the ApoE4 allele. More recent research, however, suggests that even light drinking may be harmful, promoting changes in the brain's volume and white matter.[54] Heavy consumption of alcohol is associated with many adverse health effects and should be avoided. It is also important to be aware of the amount of sugar and other carbohydrates in drinks as well as the diuretic effect of alcohol that contributes to dehydration. People who have not previously consumed alcohol should not begin drinking it for the sole purpose of Alzheimer's prevention or treatment.

Alcohol-related dementia (ARD) is cognitive impairment induced by excessive drinking over a period of time and causes functional and structural changes in the brain.[55] Symptoms are similar to Alzheimer's and worsen if alcohol consumption is not reduced. Treatment begins with cessation of alcohol intake and may include addressing withdrawal symptoms when necessary (under medical supervision) and psychological support. If abstinence is sustained, it may be possible to partially recover some of the brain's white matter, which would lead to improvements in cognition and motor skills.[56]

Artificial Ingredients
Although evidence on any particular ingredient may not be strong, there is mounting evidence that sweeteners, flavors, colors, and preservatives can have negative impacts on health, especially over the course of a lifetime. Foods made with artificial ingredients often contain chemicals that the body does not recognize as food.[57, 58] Food dyes have been linked to hyperactivity and attention-deficit/hyperactivity disorder (ADHD) in children.[59, 60] Other research suggests that food additives may alter the gut microbiota, contributing to metabolic diseases and inflammation, which potentially impact cognition and behavior.[61] See the Toxins chapter for more information on food additives.

Chocolate
Flavanols are compounds found in plants that fight inflammation and protect against cell damage caused by free radicals. Cocoa beans are high in flavanols, and research has shown that consuming a beverage high in cocoa flavanols can have beneficial effects on brain function as well as insulin resistance, blood pressure, and lipid peroxidation.[62] Consuming even a small amount of dark chocolate can help increase cerebral blood flow.[63] The darker the chocolate (at least 70 percent cacao), the greater the benefits, including better reaction time, memory, and visual-spatial awareness.[64, 65]

However, there is reason to be cautious about sources of dark chocolate, even if it is organic. A 2022 study by *Consumer Reports* found that some chocolate bars contain high levels of lead and cadmium, likely due to polluted soil and harvesting processes. Eating just an ounce a day would exceed acceptable levels of these heavy metals and potentially cause health problems. Milk chocolate is not as healthful due to its high sugar content and fewer antioxidants, but it contains lower levels of heavy metals.[66]

Foods High in Pesticides and Herbicides

Produce found in food markets may have been grown and treated with chemicals such as pesticides, herbicides, and glyphosate (commercially known as Roundup) that can cause inflammation in the body.[67] Some fruits grown outside the United States may contain DDT as well. People with the ApoE4 gene seem particularly susceptible to this pesticide and should consider consuming organic produce if it is grown outside the United States.[68, 69]

Every year, the Environmental Working Group (ewg.org) publishes a list of the Clean 15 and Dirty 12, the latter being those fruits and vegetables that contain herbicides, pesticides, or are otherwise considered less healthy. Most of the Clean 15 have thicker rinds to protect the fruit or vegetable or are less heavily sprayed. See the Toxins chapter for a broader discussion on this topic.

Fried Foods, Pastries, Sweets, Cheese, Butter, and Margarine

Overindulgence in these foods is negatively associated with heart and brain health, and both the MIND and DASH diets recommend minimizing their intake. Recent studies show that consuming ultra-processed foods is associated with cognitive decline,[70] and people with Type 2 diabetes may be at increased risk.[71, 72]

Grains

Grains are found in all cultures and include wheat, corn, rice, oats, barley, quinoa, sorghum, teff, and rye. Whole grains are almost always a healthier option than refined grains because they preserve nutrients and fiber by keeping the bran, germ, and endosperm together. The recommended amount of grain consumption ranges from over three servings per day in the MIND diet to one to two per day or fewer in more recent writings.[73] Grain consumption itself is a complex and developing subject. Consuming grains has been shown to raise blood sugar in people who may have a predisposition to diabetes. Those who have higher than normal blood glucose levels should consider limiting even whole grains. An additional consideration for those with sensitivity is the presence of gluten in grains such as wheat, spelt, barley, and rye, which can adversely affect gut health.

Salt
Excessive sodium intake can negatively affect cardiovascular health and raise blood pressure, which are both risk factors for cognitive decline.[74] The American Heart Association suggests an ideal daily limit of 1,500 mg per day and says the average American intake is around 3,400 mg. Although rare, extremely low sodium intake (less than 500 mg per day) may result in low blood sodium, which is also associated with cognitive decline.[75]

Sugar, High Glycemic Foods, and Processed Foods
Sugar has multiple effects on the body and brain and comes in many forms. Consistently ingesting sugar or having high blood sugar spikes can lead to insulin resistance, the inability of the hormone insulin to move glucose from the blood into cells, where it is used for energy. In this instance, cells throughout the body no longer respond to the normal actions of insulin, and the greater amount of refined carbohydrates and sugar that are ingested, the more resistant the cells are likely to become. Research clearly shows insulin resistance and diabetes are risk factors for Alzheimer's disease.[76] Elevated levels of blood sugar over a long period of time can cause inflammation and oxidative stress in the body.

Insulin resistance may also increase Alzheimer's risk because the same enzyme responsible for breaking down insulin also helps clear away beta amyloid in the brain.[77] Due to this relationship, it may be that the enzyme cannot effectively clear the beta amyloid in people who have high levels of insulin because the enzyme is busy breaking down the insulin. Over time, beta amyloid builds up, leading to amyloid plaques, which are a signature feature of Alzheimer's.[78]

- **Added Sugars:** Added sugars (as listed on food labels) and sugar in general have the most direct and fastest impact on blood sugar levels, so intake should be minimized. Simply checking food labels for sugar is a good first step, being aware that any ingredient ending in *-ose* (e.g., maltose, sucrose) is also a sugar. Other names for sugar include molasses, high fructose corn syrup, honey, and fruit juice concentrates. For whole, unprocessed foods, glycemic index numbers (see the following discussion) are a good resource for determining blood sugar impact.

- **Sugar Alcohols and Substitutes:**
  » Sugar alcohols are used in products including sugar-free gum and candy and provide sweetness with fewer calories than sugar. They do not generally have a large effect on blood sugar and, for some people, can be a reasonable reduced-calorie sugar substitute option. They are not necessarily healthy foods as they often have a laxative effect, can cause bowel irritation, and may still impact blood sugar. Common sugar alcohols found in foods include mannitol, sorbitol, xylitol, lactitol, isomalt, maltitol, and hydrogenated starch hydrolysates (HSH). At the very least, due to their sweetness, sugar alcohols may drive a desire for sweet foods.
  » Sugar substitutes, also known as nonnutritive sweeteners (NNS), typically have no calories and are more intensely sweet than regular sugar. They are found in beverages and processed foods and may be used in cooking and baking. While early research had been inconclusive about any ill or dangerous effects of NNS,

a 2023 study found a link to an increased risk of strokes, heart attacks, and related cardiovascular problems. The study reported, "Aspartame (NutraSweet, Equal) was linked to a higher risk of stroke, while acesulfame potassium (Sunnett, Sweet One) and sucralose (Splenda) were associated with higher coronary artery disease risk."[79] Consuming higher amounts of artificial sweeteners was also correlated with a higher risk of diabetes.[80] Monk fruit and stevia are two natural sweeteners that do not adversely impact blood sugar. They are still somewhat processed, but are perhaps better options as low calorie sugar substitutes.

- **Processed Carbohydrates:** Refined carbohydrates, including pasta, bread, breakfast cereals, packaged snacks, and crackers, can have effects on the body similar to sugar. Processing carbohydrates often involves removing the natural fiber that slows down the rate of carbohydrate absorption, which results in blood sugar rising faster than the body can manage. As a general rule, the more processed a carbohydrate, the less healthy it will be. While it is difficult to avoid these foods altogether, following a whole foods, plant-based diet can minimize consumption of them.

- **High Glycemic Foods:** High glycemic foods contain "simple" carbohydrates that raise blood sugar levels. However, not all carbohydrates are equal in terms of their impact on the body. One way to understand the effect various foods have on blood sugar levels is to learn their glycemic index (GI) and glycemic load (GL) numbers.[81] The glycemic index is a way to classify foods that contain carbohydrates and their potential for raising blood sugar. Foods with a high glycemic index would include, for example, white bread, white rice, corn chips, fruit juice, and white potatoes. Low glycemic index foods would include leafy greens and nonstarch vegetables, berries, nuts, beans, dairy, and protein. GL reflects a food's total impact on blood sugar and takes into account the total amount of carbohydrates. Watermelon, for example, is a food that has a high GL but a low GI because it contains few carbohydrates.

Unhealthy Fats (Saturated Fats and Trans Fats)
Foods with saturated fat include dairy (butter, milk, cheese, margarine), meat, tallow, and lard. Intake of saturated fats is associated with an increased risk of Alzheimer's and dementia.[82] When consumption of foods containing saturated fats is necessary, substituting a milk alternative with less saturated and trans fats is advisable. Examples include almond or oat milk instead of dairy. Medium-chain triglycerides, as mentioned earlier, are also considered saturated fats that have shorter carbon atom chains than other fats. According to a 2016 study, "medium, and possibly shorter chain, saturated fats behave differently than long-chain saturated fats and should not be judged similarly when it comes to their cardio-metabolic health effects."[83]

Beyond Nutrition: Dietary Strategies and Considerations

Caloric Intake: Personalize, Monitor, and Potentially Limit
It may be helpful to work with a doctor or registered dietician to determine the appropriate number of calories your body needs based on personal factors including height, weight, and activity level. Consuming too many calories, especially from processed foods or those high in carbohydrates, has been shown to adversely affect cognition.[84, 85, 86] Caloric restriction has been associated with reducing mild cognitive impairment (MCI) risk and lowering body mass.[87] Less visceral fat around the midsection and associated organs is associated with better cardiovascular health, lower inflammation, and lower insulin levels, which help to reduce Alzheimer's risk. It can be beneficial to the brain and body to have extended periods when the digestive system can rest. Intermittent fasting regimens have been linked to improved body-

fat composition, improved insulin sensitivity, improved cholesterol levels, lower blood pressure, and reduced inflammation, which are all possible mechanisms for reducing Alzheimer's risk.

Time-Restricted Feeding and Intermittent Fasting
A particular version of caloric restriction is fasting or restricting the period of the day that one eats. There are many versions of "fasting." The easiest is to limit the consumption of food to 12 hours during the day (e.g., 7 a.m. to 7 p.m.) and fast for the other 12 hours. Ideally, a person would finish consuming food three hours before going to sleep. For most people, this means not eating or snacking after dinner or before breakfast. Having water and unsweetened (and ideally decaffeinated) coffee and tea during fasting time is allowed. Other regimens include extending the daily fasting period up to 16, 18, or 20 hours a day or doing periodic multiday fasts.[88, 89, 90] Fasting for 14 hours per day or more is often recommended for ApoE4 carriers. Fasting is not safe for everyone, especially diabetics, and should be discussed with your doctor.

Ketogenic Diet for Those with Insulin Resistance
The ketogenic diet is a very low-carbohydrate, high-protein, and healthy-fat diet which forces the body to burn fatty acids in the form of ketones instead of glucose for energy. Shifting to a ketogenic diet may be useful for improving brain health in two ways: by correcting insulin resistance through reduction of blood glucose levels and by increasing ketone levels in the brain.

An increasing number of studies suggest that ketone levels are positively correlated with memory performance. Findings from a 2010 study indicate that low carbohydrate consumption, even in the short term, can improve memory function in older adults with an increased risk for Alzheimer's. This effect may be in part due to other mechanisms associated with ketosis, such as reduced inflammation and enhanced energy metabolism, which may also contribute to improved neurocognitive function and therefore requires further investigation.[91, 92]

The ketogenic diet has generated significant attention in recent years and derives from research on epilepsy.[93] Since the primary requirement for entering ketosis is to consume very low amounts of carbohydrates, many versions of the diet have emerged that are not nutritionally sound. A little common sense can go a long way in its application (i.e., a diet of red meat, pork rinds, and diet soda is still unhealthy even if it is "keto"). A reasonable approach would be to continue following the basic structure of the MIND diet, reduce sources of carbohydrates, and increase sources of healthy fats. Working with a healthcare professional will ensure a regimen that is appropriate.

Specific Supplements to Boost Brain Function

Supplements should be consumed under the supervision of and in consultation with a physician. Every supplement may not be necessary for every individual; where possible, a supplement will be used following testing that indicates it is needed.

- **Vitamin D3:** Low vitamin D3 levels have been linked to poor memory. Testing and supplementation may be necessary to raise levels above 55 nmol/L.[94, 95] It is suggested that vitamin D3 be combined with vitamin K2-7 (also known as menaquinone-7 or MK-7), a form of vitamin K that has health-beneficial effects in osteoporosis, cardiovascular disease, inflammation, cancer, Alzheimer's disease, diabetes, and peripheral neuropathy. These combined supplements aid in calcium absorption and utilization in the bones.[96]
- **Vitamin E:** Supplementation with certain forms of this vitamin has been shown to slow down the progression of memory loss.[97] As vitamin E is actually a set of different compounds, one should supplement with a version that has mixed tocopherols and tocotrienols.

- **Omega 3 Fatty Acids (EPA and DHA)**: These healthy fats found in cold-water fish are essential for brain function. DHA, alone or combined with EPA, has been shown to contribute to improved memory function in older adults with mild memory complaints. For optimal benefit, aim for 900 mg of DHA combined with an equal or lower amount of EPA using a fish oil supplement.[98, 99, 100]
- **B Vitamins:** This includes vitamin B12, B9 (folate), and B6. All three are essential for healthy brain function. Typically, they are taken in the form of a complete "B complex" and prescribed by your doctor based on your genetics and blood levels of homocysteine. Methylcobalamin is the preferred version of B12 due to its bioavailability.[101]

There are additional supplements that may be recommended by a physician based on an individual's lab results. Supplements often vary in their quality and ability to be absorbed by the body, and a blood test can determine if the supplement is having the desired effect.

Food Allergies, Gut Health, and Diet-Related Inflammation

Sometimes health problems result from consuming our very favorite foods, and simply removing them from our plates is all that is required to make us feel a lot better. Food can cause inflammation if one is allergic or sensitive to it, and one way to discover potential food allergies or sensitivities is to follow an elimination diet. This type of diet involves refraining completely from consuming the most common allergens, keeping a food journal to help pinpoint what changes were made and when, and recording any improvements in symptoms (such as reduced irritability, better energy, better mental focus, etc.). Common allergens include dairy, nuts, soy, wheat, foods containing gluten, eggs, and seafood. After improvements are felt for a period of time and if they seem to have stabilized, allergens may be reintroduced, one at a time, for two to three days to see what symptoms — if any — return. If there is a recurrence, those foods may be avoided in order to control those symptoms.

Another way to check for food sensitivities is for a doctor to run tests that detect reactions to a panel of different foods over days or weeks. These are immunoglobulin tests, known as IgG and IgA tests. Knowing which foods are producing an inflammatory response will allow the individual to avoid those foods, thereby reducing inflammation.

Conclusion

No two individuals are the same, and it is necessary for patients to work with their doctors to determine what dietary guidelines and supplements are most effective. Changing the way we eat is a complicated endeavor that may mean changing habits built over a lifetime or adapting recommendations for diets of different cultures. It is recommended that changes be made slowly and that health practitioners create realistic expectations with their patients. Engaging a health coach who is trained to work with clients to set health goals and make slow, steady progress toward meeting them may be helpful. Small steps that result in sustainable changes to one's lifestyle over time is the desired outcome.

2

Physical Activity

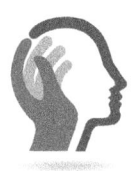

MANY HEALTH PROFESSIONALS REFER TO PHYSICAL activity and exercise as the closest thing to a wonder drug, which certainly applies to brain health. Dr. Dale Bredesen, author of *The End of Alzheimer's Program*, rates exercise as "the single most important strategy you can employ to prevent and remediate cognitive decline."[102] It is widely accepted that physical exercise positively impacts many factors that contribute to memory loss, such as improving sleep, reducing stress, and regulating blood sugar. Because brain health often reflects the overall health of the body, the World Health Organization (WHO) strongly states that regular physical activity has benefits for the brain on a molecular level, on the body's systems, and generally, on our quality of life.[103]

The body of research supporting the benefits of exercise for cognitive health is robust and growing. The benefits of exercise come directly from its ability to reduce insulin resistance, reduce inflammation, and stimulate the release of growth factors such as brain-derived neurotrophic factor (BDNF). These are proteins in the brain that impact the health, abundance, and survival of brain cells and the growth of new blood vessels in the brain. Indirectly, exercise improves mood and sleep and reduces stress and anxiety. Problems in these areas frequently cause or contribute to cognitive impairment.[104, 105]

Why Exercise Matters to the Brain

Exercise helps memory and thinking through direct and indirect means. Increasing physical activity and incorporating a healthy level of exercise into daily life directly impacts the brain and improves many other processes that enhance brain health.

The following are some of the many benefits of regular exercise for the brain:
- Promotes a strong flow of oxygen and blood to support the formation of new brain cells
- Increases BDNF
- Can increase the size of the hippocampus and prefrontal cortex
- Can support new brain cell formation
- Controls blood sugar levels
- Improves mood
- Promotes better sleep
- Reduces stress
- Reduces inflammation throughout the body
- Keeps joints and muscles limber
- Builds strength and flexibility
- Improves balance to prevent injuries
- Maintains the natural rhythm of the body's circulatory, lymph, and elimination systems
- Provides opportunities to socialize

Different Types of Exercise Have Different Benefits

The generally recommended approach to exercise for brain health is three to four sessions per week that each last 45 to 60 minutes and include a mix of aerobic workouts, strength training, and exercises for stability and flexibility.[106, 107] Raising the heart rate to the point of perspiring promotes detoxification, and keeping the heart rate elevated for about 20 minutes increases blood circulation and oxygenation.[108]

Even sports like table tennis can have a striking impact on cognitive function.[109]

A 2021 study showed that high levels of exercise do the most to reduce Alzheimer's risk, but even light exercise lowers risk.[110] A population study of Swedish twins also showed that regular exercise in midlife — even light exercise such as gardening or walking — may reduce the incidence of dementia in older adulthood.[111]

OSE vs. CSE Exercise
Going even further, recent research has looked at exercise that requires active decision-making and adaptability in unpredictable environments with reactions to randomly occurring stimuli (called OSE for "open-skill environments") versus repetitive activities in more controlled environments (CSE, or "closed-skill environments"). A 2023 study showed that OSE activities (such as basketball, tennis, and handball) have a more beneficial impact on cognitive health than CSE activities (such as swimming laps, cycling, running, or shooting).[112] Those engaging in the former activities exhibited better executive functioning and had higher BDNF levels.

Aerobic Exercise
Aerobic exercise is any physical activity that increases heart rate and improves cardiovascular endurance. It typically involves continuous, rhythmic movements of large muscle groups, such as walking, running, cycling, or swimming. Aerobic exercise keeps the body's systems moving and functioning well by strengthening the heart and lungs, boosting stamina, circulating oxygen and other nutrients, and eliminating waste and toxins.

Research consistently shows that aerobic exercise has many benefits for the brain, including increasing the size of the hippocampus, a key brain region associated with memory and learning, generating new blood vessels, raising levels of BDNF, and increasing the development of new neurons.[113, 114] Regular aerobic activity can enhance cognitive function and promote neuroplasticity in both older and younger adults. A 2019 study of 132 adults between the ages of 20 and 67 showed an improvement in executive function and an increase in gray matter, reflected in the thickening of the frontal cortex.[115]

What may be most important is the role that aerobic exercise plays in the prevention of cognitive decline. A meta-analysis of more than 30,000 older adults over five years found that those who engaged in higher levels of aerobic exercise were 38 percent less likely to experience cognitive decline. Even those study participants who reported doing low to moderate levels of physical exercise had a 35 percent reduced risk of cognitive decline.[116] The findings suggest that aerobic activity may help to stave off brain aging and improve overall brain performance.[117]

Approximately 150 minutes of total exercise per week, or an average of 30 minutes per day, is recommended. When doing aerobic exercise, intensity plays a role. Our bodies will not experience the benefits if we just amble along or cycle at a level that isn't challenging. Walk with intention, as if you are late to meet someone, and be as consistent as possible with your exercise routine. Consult with a physical fitness trainer or your doctor for safe guidelines.

HIIT Training

High-intensity interval training (HIIT), where one exercises at high intensity for a short period followed by lower intensity exercise or brief rest, has been shown to have positive effects on fitness and cognition. A 2023 study has shown that just six minutes of HIIT increases BDNF and can delay the onset of Alzheimer's disease.[118]

HIIT has been shown to improve cognition and psychological well-being in children and young adults and continues to support brain health into middle age and beyond. A 2021 review studied people aged 19 to 40 who did HIIT for 11 minutes and assessed three areas of cognitive function: inhibition (the ability to restrain automatic responses during cognitive processing), working memory (the capacity to store and process temporary information), and cognitive flexibility. Consistent positive effects were seen in the first two categories.[119] In another study of people in their 60s and 70s, participants were divided into one of three groups: The first completed 40-minute HIIT workouts three times a week; the second performed 30 to 39 minutes of moderately intense cycling; and the third had eight sessions of resistance training. Those in the HIIT group had better cardiorespiratory fitness and cognitive flexibility compared to the other two groups. They also demonstrated more cognitive flexibility on the Stroop Test, a set of tasks that measure attention and processing speed.[120]

Strength Training
A 2010 study of women 65 to 75 years of age who received strength training once or twice a week over 12 months showed improved executive cognitive functioning, especially in the areas of selective attention and conflict resolution.[121] Six months of high-intensity resistance exercise was also shown to have beneficial effects on cognition in those with mild cognitive impairment, including protection from hippocampal volume loss up to a year post-training.[122] Another small study showed that resistance training and exercise led not only to functional brain changes in the frontal lobe, thereby improving executive function, but also to lower white matter atrophy and smaller white matter lesion volumes.[123] More information on the biological processes underlying resistance training can be found in a narrative review by Zunner, Wachsmuth, et al.[124] The results of these studies point to the importance of resistance training as part of a weekly exercise routine.

Yoga and Pilates
Practices such as yoga, Pilates, and meditation are recognized as safe techniques that may have beneficial effects on cognitive function and improve health in older adults at risk for cognitive decline. For example, when combined with a regular exercise program, yoga can improve cardiovascular health by lowering blood pressure and resting heart rate

and improve 10-year cardiovascular risk.[125] Yoga has also been shown to reduce levels of hemoglobin A1c (a measure of blood sugar)[126] and improve heart rate variability.[127] Yoga improves mental well-being, cognitive abilities, depression, and mood[128] and the functioning of parts of the brain, including the hippocampus, amygdala, prefrontal cortex, and cingulate cortex.[129] A review of the literature suggests positive evidence that yoga-based interventions improve attention, executive function, and memory compared to active controls among the elderly.[130]

Pilates has also been shown to improve cognition in older adults. A study of Spanish women over age 60 showed that verbal fluency, executive function, lower body strength, and functional flexibility improved after a 12-week training program of Pilates exercises.[131] Pilates was shown to be more effective than muscular exercises in maintaining women's general functional condition as they age. In a separate study, elderly subjects who participated in two Pilates classes a week for 13 weeks improved in agility, flexibility, endurance, and attention and concentration.[132]

Tai Chi/Qigong

Qigong and a subtype of Qigong called Tai Chi are ancient practices that engage body and mind. Qigong consists of slow and gentle movements regulated with breath. Tai Chi is based in martial arts and has prescribed circular movements and pelvic rotations coordinated with the breath in a state of relaxation and repeated in a specific sequence. Both practices help to maintain strength, flexibility, and balance and are meant to unblock energy channels in the body and promote self-healing. These practices have also been linked to better cognition in older adults.[133]

Many studies have looked at the effects of Tai Chi practice on cognition, especially because it is exercise accessible to people of all ages. Tai Chi has been shown to improve working memory,[134] verbal memory,[135] and memory retrieval processes.[136] A study of older adults with MCI and Type 2 diabetes showed that Tai Chi was more effective than fitness walking in improving global cognitive function.[137]

Systematic reviews of studies and randomized controlled trials looking at the cognitive benefits of Tai Chi suggest that it "may improve memory and cognition via increased regional brain activity, large-scale network functional connectivity, and regional grey matter volume."[138]

A 2023 study looked at Qigong and cognition through brain imaging studies. Eighteen studies from 11 randomized controlled trials showed that Qigong induced structural and functional changes in various brain regions, many of which impact memory. Changes in the prefrontal cortex and hippocampus likely contributed to positive changes in cognition, and these were consistent for both the healthy and cognitively impaired populations.[139]

While Qigong is often practiced outdoors, indoor classes were used in a study that looked at not only the effects of Qigong on cognitive function but also the mechanisms by which they were achieved. Specifically, improvements were seen in processing speed and sustained attention with associated increases in hippocampal volume and reduced peripheral interleukin-6 (IL-6) levels (a marker of inflammation).[140]

Starting an Exercise Program

Everyone's ability to exercise is different, and it is important to increase to optimal levels slowly and do so with a doctor's guidance. There is little value in abruptly increasing exercise levels and risking injury.[141] Guidelines for the amounts of recommended activity are in the following lists.

Type of Exercise

AEROBIC OR CARDIO
2–3 times per week
- Running, biking, hiking, brisk walking
- Swimming, water aerobics
- Rowing, kayaking, paddling
- Circuit training
- Dancing, Zumba

Pay close attention to any pain, and scale back when necessary. There is no need to be a marathoner to gain the benefits of cardio.

HIIT (HIGH-INTENSITY INTERVAL TRAINING)
Add in HIIT-style workouts to a cardio program.
- Spin class
- Alternate jogging and sprinting

These workouts are characterized by short bursts of high-intensity exercise followed by lower intensity rest periods.

RESISTANCE OR STRENGTH TRAINING
2 times per week (if tolerated)
- Circuit machines (a good place to start since they reduce risk of injury)
- Body-weight exercise
- Free weights
- Resistance bands

Target the eight main muscle groups (knee extension and flexion; abdomen and back muscles; rotation; upper back; arm muscles; press bench for lower extremity muscles).

STABILITY/FLEXIBILITY/MIND-BODY
Beneficial on rest days from cardio/weights, this type of exercise can be one part of a complete fitness program.

- Yoga
- Tai Chi
- Pilates
- Qigong

These workouts help to avoid injuries, keep the body ready for cardio and strength workouts, and contribute to better brain health on their own.

Self-Assessment and Planning

In any fitness program, it is important to begin by setting small, measurable goals that build confidence. The table below is one way to track various types of exercise, duration, and frequency of exercise per week. Set objectives for the coming week that reflect a modest and attainable increase over the previous week's goals.

Type of Exercise	Last Week		Next Week	
	Minutes/ week	Times/ week	Minutes/ week	Times/ week
Aerobic/ cardio				
HIIT				
Resistance/ strength				
Mind-body/ stability				
Total				

Here are some helpful suggestions for those who are beginning an exercise program:
- Begin gradually by walking for 15 minutes/day and increasing over time to one hour to build endurance.
- Choose activities that raise heart rate and generate perspiration.
- Learn a new activity like ballroom dancing, bike riding, or martial arts.
- Create a workout space and accountability system: Join a gym, exercise with a friend, or work with a trainer to stay motivated.
- Do aerobic exercise several days a week, working up to 30 to 45 minutes/day.
- Try strength training, covering all of the major muscle groups, 2 to 3 times/week.
- Try exercise apps or other technology tools:
  » Running, walking, and biking apps such as MapMyRun, MyFitnessPal, and Wahoo Fitness
  » Wearable fitness devices that track heart rate, activity, and distance, such as chest strap monitors, Apple Watch, Fitbit devices, Oura Ring, and others
  » Live and on-demand fitness classes offered by exercise equipment manufacturers such as Peleton, NordicTrack, Fitness Blender, or BowFlex
- Consider working with a professional for one or more sessions to develop a personalized workout plan that addresses individual fitness levels, physical limitations, and personal goals.

Conclusion

When people ask what the most important thing they can do to care for their brains is, regular physical activity tops the list. Not only does exercise keep every system in the body moving and functioning optimally, it also provides more oxygen for the brain, increases BDNF, decreases stress, and helps us to manage weight and blood sugar.

Each of us enjoys different sports and ways of moving our bodies; finding those favorites and doing them regularly, especially with a friend, increases the likelihood of making exercise a regular part of life. Including strength training and activities that test and improve balance will also keep bones healthy and prevent falls. Staying active and flexible as we age increases the likelihood of engaging in the activities we most enjoy with friends and family we care about.

3

Mental Stimulation

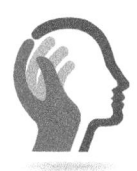

IT MAY SEEM OBVIOUS THAT KEEPING ourselves mentally stimulated is good for our brains. However, as we age, it is not uncommon for people to have developed habits like watching television or scrolling through social media that are either passive activities or that require little mental concentration. In addition, repeating the same ways we do things — often on autopilot, such as driving the same route to a familiar destination — doesn't challenge the brain. Growing new neuronal synapses and improving brain function are often associated with learning new skills and activities such as taking up a new instrument or language, using new technology, or learning a new dance.[142] This is what keeps our brain stimulated and healthy.

Defining Mental Stimulation

Clinical psychologists Linda Clare and Robert T. Woods categorized mental stimulation interventions into three types based on the mode of delivery and the goals of the intervention: cognitive stimulation, cognitive rehabilitation, and cognitive training.[143] Cognitive stimulation refers to more general activities such as group discussions, reading, or list memorization. Cognitive rehabilitation refers to targeted programs designed to help individuals regain function in their daily lives, but not improve cognition per se. Cognitive training seeks to improve cognition and memory and is focused on such tasks as attention or problem-solving with the expectation that practice has the potential to maintain or improve functioning in the given cognitive domain. All three types of mental stimulation can effectively improve brain health or quality of life; it is appropriate to consider personal goals and what the best methods are to achieve them.

Support for the potential role of mentally stimulating activities in preventing or mitigating cognitive decline comes from animal studies, observational studies in humans, and to a lesser extent, randomized clinical trials.[144] Observational studies have found that high levels of participation in mentally stimulating leisure activities such as traveling, reading, playing games such as checkers and cards, and doing crossword puzzles were helpful in maintaining cognition levels.[145]

Clinical trials have also shown the effectiveness of mentally stimulating activities for improving cognitive function in specific tasks for which subjects were trained. The FINGER study, a seminal multi-domain lifestyle study, used cognitive training in addition to nutrition and exercise to improve cognition in over 1,200 men and women. The treatment group improved in complex memory, executive functioning, and processing speed compared to the control group.[146] In addition, Posit Science (brainhq.com) has conducted research to show that cognition was improved by playing their brain games, especially Double Decision and Hawkeye.[147]

Cognitive improvement has been attributed to several factors: building cognitive reserve,[148] improving vascular health, and managing stress. (See the chapters on Prolonged Stress and Physical and Emotional Trauma for references to related research.) Cognitive reserve is a measure of the resilience of the brain and the degree of its susceptibility to age-related brain changes or pathology associated with Alzheimer's disease. Researchers have suggested that cognitive reserve may help to explain why individuals with similar risk factors for dementia and physiological changes in the brain have widely varied cognitive conditions. Cognitive reserve is correlated with higher education and occupational levels and participation in leisure activities in which neurons, synapses, and blood vessels have been expanded over a long period of time.[149] People with greater cognitive reserve are often able to withstand the pathology of dementia longer before their cognitive function declines but experience more rapid decline once a diagnosis is made.[150]

Keeping the Mind Active

Activities that use several senses, involve the body, and engage the mind generally result in greater health benefits for the brain.

Practical suggestions:
- Stay curious: Read books, visit museums, attend movies and other cultural events.
- Continue learning by taking classes on topics of special interest.
- Play games that exercise the brain:
  » Try the brain challenges from Posit Science (brainhq.com), specifically Hawkeye and Double Decision games.
  » Play cards, chess, or board games; do puzzles or brain teasers.
- Listen to, play, or compose music: Research has shown that listening to music can reduce anxiety and blood pressure while also improving sleep quality, mental alertness, and memory.[151, 152]
- Combine mental, social, and physical challenges: Try using the opposite hand when eating or brushing your teeth, for example.
- Learn new things or reengage with previous interests:
  » Take a series of classes or pursue a degree: Research indicates that more education provides greater protection against cognitive decline.
  » Learn a language or return to a language you used to know.

- » Learn a musical instrument or return to an instrument you used to play.
- » Engage more deeply in hobbies and seek out new activities.
- Write in a journal, create fictional stories, start a blog.
- Find an occupation that gives meaning and purpose.
- Be social (but not on social media).
- Join a club of interest: books, culture, chess, cards, faith-based or other.

Conclusion

It is not surprising that keeping our minds active and engaged throughout life helps to ward off memory loss and dementia. Even if we didn't enjoy school and don't have a college degree, it's never too late to take a class, in person or online, or try a new hobby or pastime, especially with a friend or someone whose company we enjoy. Even people who aren't very social play games on a phone or computer that challenge the mind. Mental stimulation is just one of the many lifestyle factors we want to foster to keep our brains sharp as we age.

4

Social Interaction

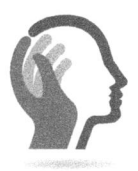

HUMAN BEINGS ARE SOCIAL CREATURES, and our overall well-being depends on social connection. Staying socially active also contributes to health and longevity. Beyond the stigma of loneliness, being isolated or lacking a support system has important evolutionary implications. As a "tribal" species, our bodies and minds require regular human connection as much as food and water. From the perspective of our earliest ancestors, it was more dangerous to our survival to be left alone and vulnerable than it was to miss a meal. Addressing isolation and building the necessary support networks should be part of a comprehensive prevention or treatment plan for anyone concerned with dementia.

Why Social Interaction Matters

Research shows that social isolation is one of the strongest predictors of chronic disease. It is as dangerous to be lonely in our lives as it is to smoke 15 cigarettes per day, and twice as dangerous as being obese.[153] In fact, based on the same study that followed over 300,000 people for 7.5 years, those most isolated have a 50 percent higher chance of dying early than those who are not. More specifically, being isolated dramatically increases the chances of developing heart disease, stroke, cancer, and dementia.

Despite the growing presence of social media and similar "connection" technology, many people feel they lack support in their lives. Upwards of 40 percent of our population (and 43 percent of seniors) report feeling lonely or isolated, double what it was in the 1980s.[154] Much of this is due to societal changes in family structure, with many more single-person households and fewer traditional nuclear families. Few predicted that social isolation would take such a major toll on health.

Many studies have linked social isolation to developing dementia.[155] Research shows that the rate of cognitive decline was slower by an average of 70 percent in people who were frequently socially active as compared to people who were infrequently socially active. These effects, it seems, become even more pronounced after age 70.[156] A prospective cohort study in 2014 followed 1,461 subjects over 20 years who were evaluated biannually. Data on their engagement in 10 leisure and social activities was collected at baseline and at the 10-year follow-up visit for 805 subjects. After adjusting for age, gender, educational level, diabetes, stroke, and depression, results suggest a significant association between a decrease in leisure and social activities during old age and risk of dementia.[157]

Isolation may play a role for both patient and caregiver. Research shows that there is a 49 percent higher likelihood for both groups of developing dementia after 10 years of living with little social interaction.[158] The experience of helping to care for a loved one is itself a uniquely isolating experience that deserves considerable attention. A recent study found that spouse caregivers were six times more likely to develop dementia.[159] This may be because the caregiver is living a lifestyle similar to that of the person with dementia: potentially poor sleep, little exercise, less social interaction, higher stress level, and so on.

Social isolation is a broader societal issue. During the COVID pandemic, we learned that it became a matter of life and death. Stuck in houses, apartments or long-term care facilities, many elders did not have in-person contact with their families for months and perhaps years. Older adults living alone today may not have children or may live far away from their loved ones. As the years go by, friends and neighbors pass or move away; these people had looked out for one another. Isolation can be especially worrisome for people who experience forgetfulness and may be at the beginning stages of cognitive decline because it tends to exacerbate the disease.[160]

Creating a More Connected Life

Making new connections is important at every stage of life. What works for one person may not be comfortable for another. Here are some suggestions:
- Set a goal of making at least one new friend every few months.
- Engage in sports, games, and activities you enjoy.
- Volunteer for an organization or cause you believe in.
- Maintain memberships in social clubs and/or religious groups.
- Nurture close friendships and family relationships.
- Get to know your neighbors.
- Schedule and participate in social events.
- Set up a regular check-in by phone or in person with someone you like and trust.

Conclusion

Keeping older adults in our sights and engaging them at senior centers, during family and celebratory events, and in groups with others who share similar interests will keep their minds engaged and lessen feelings of isolation. People who are introverts or prefer to spend time alone still benefit from periodic interactions with friends or relatives. The research is clear that isolation is a strong risk factor for dementia, and regularly checking in with elders ensures they are physically and medically safe and have contact with people who care about them.

5

Sleep and Breathing

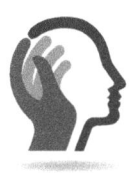

OUR BRAINS REQUIRE OXYGEN, DETOXIFICATION, and memory consolidation to survive and stay healthy. We take about 20,000 breaths every day, one roughly every four seconds, and it is generally recommended that we sleep an average of seven to eight hours a night. Even seemingly minor issues with these essential functions can develop into more significant problems over time, notably cognitive decline and dementia. This chapter focuses on the importance of breathing and sleep, how dysfunction can affect the brain, methods for identifying problems, and practical steps to ensure and create optimal function.

The Importance of Quality Breathing and Sleep in Preventing Dementia

Optimal health depends on quality breathing and sleep. Even one night of poor sleep or sleep-disordered breathing can result in episodes of oxygen desaturation (drop in oxygen levels) and an increase in inflammation. Many nights of multiple events over days, months, and years plant the seeds for chronic inflammation and lead to poor brain health. Improvements in breathing, air quality, and sleep quality will likely result in improvements in overall health, and the reality is that most people have room for improvement in these areas.

While everyone knows brain damage or death will result from a lack of oxygen, very few people — even professionals — know that less acute but chronic oxygen deprivation can have a major impact on the body. Breathing polluted or low-quality air over time can harm the brain, and disrupted sleep from poor breathing or other causes damages sleep architecture (frequency of awakening, inability to go back to sleep, amount of deep sleep and REM sleep, etc.), which inhibits detoxification and memory consolidation. Research has identified dementia as a common symptom of oxygen deprivation and sleep disturbances, especially with obstructive sleep apnea (OSA).[161, 162]

A Lifetime of Breathing and Sleep

Although dementia occurs primarily in the elderly, risk factors can begin to develop as early as childhood. For example, mouth breathing can cause abnormal facial and dental development and poor sleeping habits that interfere with growth and academic performance. The damage may present during childhood as neurobehavioral and neurocognitive disorders, often resulting in a misdiagnosis of ADHD.[163] However, later in life, consequences extend to substantially increased risk of cancer, diabetes, stroke, heart disease, cardiac mortality, and dementia.[164, 165, 166] In adulthood, mouth breathing may cause poor oxygen concentration in the bloodstream, which in turn may lead to high blood pressure, heart problems, and sleep apnea, all risk factors for dementia. The harm is cumulative over a lifetime, and it is therefore crucial to pay attention to seemingly minor issues with sleep and breathing from an early age and as they arise.

Damage from Reduced Oxygen Levels
Repeated curtailment of air intake desaturates the blood, reducing the amount of oxygen the blood carries, and creates hypoxia, a deficiency in oxygen in the tissues. Hypoxia diminishes and distorts cellular

activity and effectiveness throughout the body, impacting normal brain development in children and brain cell replacement and brain function in adults.[167]

Poor Sleep Quality Damage
When the healthy sequence of sleep states is disturbed, the body cannot execute the essential processes during each of those stages, particularly detoxification and memory consolidation. According to Maiken Nedergaard, MD, DMSc, a leader in sleep research from the University of Rochester, glial cells shrink during the night, allowing cerebrospinal fluid to figuratively "wash the brain" and carry away waste products. But this housekeeping function of the brain, called the glymphatic system, can take place efficiently only during deep NREM sleep, and it requires at least 20 percent of total sleep time per night.[168] The process removes beta amyloid and tau proteins, which play significant roles in Alzheimer's pathology; robbing the brain of deep sleep may contribute to the buildup of these proteins in the Alzheimer's-affected brain.[169] Poor sleep also disrupts memory consolidation, another vital sleep process in which new memories are stored and unused information is pruned away. Without this memory consolidation process, memory recall diminishes over time.[170]

Secondary Sleep Effects
Why are these primary sleep and breathing disruptions so often unrecognized, undiagnosed as problematic, and consequently untreated? Very few people are aware that hypoxia and fragmented sleep architecture produce the following secondary effects that can cause or contribute to dementia symptoms:
- **Weakened blood-brain barrier**: A weakness in the blood-brain barrier allows an increase in toxins and a buildup of the brain's toxic load.[171]
- **Hardening of arteries**: Oxygen deprivation causes the tissues in the lining of the blood vessels to stiffen, which prevents the vessels

from expanding enough to carry adequate nutrition throughout the body.
- **Increased oxidative stress:** Hypoxia and sleep disturbances increase oxidative stress, generating more free radicals than the body can neutralize and thus leading to DNA damage.[172]
- **Systemic inflammation:** Hypoxia and disturbed sleep architecture create inflammation throughout the body, which leads to premature aging and mental and physical deterioration.[173]
- **Disrupted diet control:** A lack of sleep disrupts the hunger and satiety hormones, ghrelin and leptin, and without the natural signals for when to eat and stop eating, it is common to overeat. Decreased willpower also results from decreased sleep and contributes to this effect.[174]
- **Diminished cognitive ability:** Lack of sleep results in diminished cognitive ability. After only one night, a buildup of beta amyloid can be detected, which is also typically seen in people with Alzheimer's disease.[175]

Breathing and Airway Problems

Neither the public nor the professional community — even dentists, neurologists, pulmonologists, and ENT specialists — is equipped with the necessary training and education to understand the severe damage caused by dysfunctional breathing patterns, especially during sleep. Fortunately, the consequences of airway problems can be alleviated with proper treatment and even dramatically reversed in some cases.[176, 177] CPAP and oral appliance therapy can reverse many deficits, and many more options are becoming available. One study from The Center for Cognitive Neuroscience in Italy was highly encouraging. Researchers identified patients suffering from OSA who had decreased gray matter volume in specific cerebral regions (the frontal and hippocampal regions) and deficits in executive functioning and short-term memory. These structural deficits were reversed after CPAP therapy, as were the functional and memory problems.[178] The option to treat remains available long after the breathing problem begins, in many cases well into the last third of life.

An obstructed airway also impedes optimal breathing, and the cause may be environmental factors, asthma, or a physical obstruction, either from birth or injury (e.g., a broken nose). Airway function can be mapped on a spectrum of obstruction:[179]

- **Zero blockage:** Breathing through the nose is easy, free, and full. Cells of the body are fully oxygenated.
- **Mouth breathing:** Breathing through the nose is mildly difficult to impossible, so the person breathes through the mouth, often when awake and asleep. This may occur for a part or all of the night and makes the air intake dry and interferes with sound sleep.
- **Snoring:** Snoring occurs when both nose and mouth breathing are compromised, and the membranes and structures of the airways vibrate with the pressure of air being forced through narrowed channels.
- **Upper airway resistance syndrome (UARS) and hypopnea:** These conditions are characterized by the increased effort required for inhaling without instances of full blockage (apneas). Symptoms include sleepiness, and the harm/severity of effects can range from snoring to OSA.
- **Obstructive sleep apnea (OSA):** OSA occurs when the airway is completely obstructed for 10 seconds or more at a time, causing intermittent nocturnal oxygen deprivation. A gasp reflex follows, pulling the brain up out of deep REM and NREM sleep and thus disrupting sleep architecture, sometimes hundreds of times a night.[180]

The Basics of Sleep

Sleep has many components and is therefore complex. The body relies on patterns to get asleep, stay asleep, and perform recovery and maintenance processes while asleep. This section gives a high-level overview of some significant sleep concepts to lay the foundation for discussing sleep problems and how they harm the brain. The first two sections below, the Daily Sleep/Wake Cycle and Sleep Architecture, are the sleep patterns; the second two sections, Memory Consolidation and Detoxification, are critical sleep processes for brain health.

Daily Sleep/Wake Cycle
The daily cycle of sleeping and being awake is controlled by two complementary forces that should be synchronized: circadian rhythm and sleep pressure. The circadian rhythm, a roughly 24-hour cycle, powers wakefulness and peaks in the early afternoon. The body sets this internal clock using routine external cues like daylight or eating. Sleep pressure creates sleepiness and results from the buildup of adenosine throughout the day and its clearance during the night. Maximum wakefulness occurs when the circadian rhythm is peaking and sleep pressure is low.

Sleep Architecture
The two major stage categories of sleep are REM (rapid eye movement) and NREM (non-rapid eye movement). The stages occur in cycles, with NREM weighted toward the beginning of the night and REM weighted more toward the end. Consequently, going to bed later than usual diminishes NREM, and waking up earlier reduces REM. Each stage serves many purposes. At a high level, REM sleep strengthens connections in the brain, and NREM prunes away unused connections. Deep NREM sleep is essential because it is when the glymphatic system activates.

Memory Consolidation
Memory consolidation is the nightly process of strengthening new memories and pruning away unused information. As discussed above,

both processes occur during different sleep stages, and they are both required for a healthy brain.

Detoxification Through the Glymphatic System
As previously discussed, the brain detoxification system activates during NREM deep sleep and functionally washes the brain, cleaning away the hallmark Alzheimer's protein amyloid beta.

Sleep Problems as We Age

Several issues develop as people age and may provide the basis for sleep quality and duration generally decreasing throughout life. These may impact sleep quality and duration and, therefore, brain health.

Brain Atrophy
Brains atrophy as people age, and research has shown that one of the first areas of the brain to weaken is that which helps generate sleep. The more severe the deterioration in that area, the more deep sleep loss a person experiences.[181]

Creeping Circadian Rhythm
The circadian rhythm of older people can creep forward as they age, resulting in earlier bedtimes, misaligned sleep/wake cycles, and sleep disruption. Napping and a downshifting in melatonin release also contributes to this phenomenon.

Deep Sleep Decline
Deep NREM sleep declines during aging, beginning in the late 20s and early 30s. By the mid to late 40s, 60 to 70 percent of deep sleep has eroded, and 80 to 90 percent is gone by age 70.[182]

Insomnia

People with insomnia have trouble falling asleep and/or staying asleep, which causes significant daytime impairment and dissatisfaction with their amount of sleep. Insomnia is not the same as sleep deprivation in that it is characterized by the inability to sleep even when there is ample opportunity. A diagnosis of insomnia is based on having sleep issues three nights per week that are not attributable to other mental health issues.

Sleep Deprivation

People with sleep deprivation are considered to have the ability to sleep but not take or have the opportunity to sleep. Long-term sleep deprivation has similar effects to insomnia. When we have one night of poor sleep, we may be able to make it up, but a period of insufficient sleep can have more profound effects on the body in terms of metabolic dysregulation[183] and the brain.[184]

Sleep Fragmentation

Octogenarians have less than 70 to 80 percent sleep efficiency, meaning during eight hours in bed, they spend over two hours awake. In well-controlled studies, lower sleep efficiency translates to less energy, a greater likelihood of depression, higher mortality risk, lower cognitive functioning, and worse physical health.[185]

It is also important to note that the quality of sleep and its effectiveness can be significantly diminished without being a diagnosable clinical issue. Sleep is similar to other facets of health in that one is not simply getting good or bad sleep; there is a spectrum of sleep quality. In pursuit of health, optimizing sleep, especially as one ages, can be one of the simplest and most important things to improve.

How to Improve Sleep and Breathing over a Lifetime

It is difficult to know if we have good sleep health. While we can know if we are eating poorly or not getting enough exercise, we do not know how we sleep unless we have a sleep study or wear a device that monitors our sleep (and in some cases, the data is not reliable). Sleep and sleep breathing problems can go unrecognized and untreated for years. These hidden problems lead to chronic problems decades later.

Childhood
Children need sufficient quality sleep for brain development and learning. A child's poor sleep may present as hyperactivity and poor attention (think ADHD), a craving for sugary foods, chronic ear infections, allergies, or bed-wetting. What happens in childhood does not stay in childhood, and so it is the ideal time to recognize and treat the problem.

Once a breathing problem is recognized, early intervention to open and strengthen the airway is highly recommended because adequate oxygen and detoxifying capabilities can have such an enormous impact on the development of the brain and the body. Many approaches and interventions have proven highly effective in particular cases, including breastfeeding,[186] adenotonsillectomy (removal of tonsils and adenoids),[187] rapid palate expansion to increase airway space and decrease nasal resistance,[188] allergy treatments,[189, 190] myofunctional therapy to promote proper tongue position for improved breathing,[191] and occupational therapy.[192]

Adulthood
Fortunately, we are coming to understand that while an airway sleep disorder is a significant problem, it is also usually correctable. This is a reason for real hope for adults suffering from many associated conditions long considered intractable, including dementia. Often a

partner will complain about their mate snoring, gasping for air, or otherwise making it difficult to sleep next to them, or an individual will experience extreme fatigue and go to their doctor for help.

Identifying Airway and Hypoxia Problems
The first step to improving cognition is to assess if there is a problem with breathing during sleep. Review the following indicators to see if any are experienced or exhibited.

Symptoms that Relate to Airway Sleep Disorders and Potential Neurocognitive Risk
- Foggy brain
- Memory loss
- Weight gain
- Daytime sleepiness
- Morning headache
- Chronic pain
- Difficulty concentrating and focusing
- Nocturia (multiple urinations per night)
- Cannot breathe well through the nose
- Allergies
- Allergic shiners (dark circles caused by nasal congestion)
- Asthma
- Carbohydrate cravings
- Chronic periodontal disease
- Occlusion
- Snoring/disturbed sleep:
    » Frequent arousals
    » Gasping
    » Restless legs
- Tongue enlargement:
    » Can't see back of throat when mouth is open

- » Can't touch back of front teeth with mouth open wide
- » Scalloped edges
- Taking medications for:
  - » Sleep or pain
  - » Blood pressure or lipidemia
  - » Thyroid or diabetes

If these indicators are present in significant numbers or intensity, the following steps may be taken to determine if sleep and breathing are impaired:
- Take the STOP-Bang sleep test online (http://www.stopbang.ca/osa/screening.php).
- Fill out an Epworth Sleepiness questionnaire (https://www.mdapp.co/epworth-sleepiness-scale-calculator-201/).
- Ask your bed partner or caregiver if you snore or ever stop breathing.
- Ask yourself:
  - » "Do I have a poor memory or difficulty concentrating?"
  - » "Do I clench or grind my teeth at night?"
- Schedule a sleep study: If the answers to all these questions suggest sleep and airway disorders are a problem, make an appointment for a sleep study with a sleep physician, ear-nose-throat (ENT) specialist, or dentist trained in diagnosing and treating airway, sleep, and breathing problems.

Taking Action

There are many ways to improve the quality of breathing and sleeping. This section covers sleep testing basics as well as practical tips for better breathing and sleep hygiene.

Sleep Testing

A sleep test is the only fully reliable way to understand sleep and possible issues. Whether done at home or in a lab, every sleep test measures how often and to what degree sleep is disturbed. The report may describe the pattern of disturbance as "intermittent hypoxia" and/or "disturbed sleep architecture," which means the person failed to get adequate amounts of REM or stage 3 NREM, the deepest levels of restorative sleep. The results of a sleep study can be surprising. For example, adults with snoring, resistive breathing, and apnea may wake up hundreds of times in a single night without even knowing it. The only evidence may be feeling groggy and fuzzy in the morning. For this reason, if indicators in the previous section are present, a sleep study is indicated even if sleep quality and breathing are reported to be fine.

Better Breathing
Airway and breathing health may be improved by:
- Shedding excess weight by reducing or eliminating dairy, sugar, and gluten, for example, as well as foods that cause sensitivities or allergic reactions.
- Sleeping in a more upright position.
- Sleeping appliances to open airways. There are custom devices as well as those available over the counter. Custom devices are more expensive; however, 50 to 85 percent of bite plates/night guards for preventing teeth grinding have been shown by research to make the problem *worse* by narrowing or closing the airway, so make sure to purchase one designed for opening the airway, not just grinding.

Improved Sleep Hygiene

This section includes a list of tips, techniques, and tools that may help increase the quality and quantity of sleep. These options are not prescriptive, and each one will not be right for everyone. Additionally, they should be implemented one at a time to see what works; it is crucial to monitor whether something may improve or diminish your sleep quality. The goal here is to identify a wide range of options and for each person to choose what is most appropriate for them.

Waking Up
- Wake up and go to sleep at the same time every day. Your body craves a routine to normalize the sleep pressure and circadian rhythm cycles.
- Consider using a sleep tracker. Getting data on your sleep can help cut through the illusion that you're sleeping well and provide a tool for experimenting with sleep-promoting habits. Even your phone can be a sleep tracker, and many fitness trackers or smartwatches have sleep-tracking capabilities. High-quality sleep trackers include the WHOOP biosensor, Oura Ring, Fitbit, and Apple Watch. Merely knowing the amount of time you are asleep is extremely useful in the process of trying to get better sleep. You may be surprised by how much of the night you are awake without realizing it. *Note: Having a phone or smartwatch in bed with you may detract from sound sleep. In this case, consider using this type of tracker for a week to understand sleep patterns and then remove the electronic device from the bedroom.*

During the Day
- Exercise! Sleep helps improve exercise, and exercise helps improve sleep. It even creates adenosine, which controls sleep pressure. It is generally recommended that strenuous exercise be avoided a couple of hours before bedtime.
- Monitor caffeine intake later in the day. Consider stopping caffeine intake up to 14 hours before bedtime. Caffeine has a half-life of 6 hours, so 25 percent of the caffeine you consume is still in your system 12 hours later. *Note: Caffeine metabolism varies widely in individuals.*
- Be aware of long naps. Adenosine, your body's signal to fall asleep, builds up throughout the day and gets depleted during sleep. Some of the critical buildup of adenosine will be removed if you nap, and your natural bedtime will be delayed. Instead, stay awake throughout the day and allow yourself an earlier bedtime.

- Get sunlight during the day. Your body's circadian rhythm depends on sunlight exposure to function optimally, so be sure to get sunlight during the daylight hours in addition to limiting light before bed. Sunlight or even brighter lights at home early in the day will help you feel more awake.

Preparing for Sleep
- Avoid food three hours before bedtime. Eating and digestion can raise core body temperature, which impairs sleep, and lying down while full can increase the incidence of acid reflux at night.
- Lessen exposure to bright light. To start sending your body sleep signals:
  » Turn off screens one to two hours before retiring at night.
  » Consider using "blue blocker" glasses and night mode on devices to limit exposure to blue light, as it appears to disrupt melatonin in the body.[193]
  » Dim the lights or turn off half the lights 90 minutes before bed. Some people even use red light bulbs or smart light bulbs to limit blue light before bedtime.
- Begin the relaxation process before bed:
  » Remove all anxiety and excitement-inducing stimuli (phones, video games, or watching or reading the news).
  » Write in a journal. Some people report that writing down three things they are grateful for before bed helps them sleep well and creates a sense of peace.
  » Meditate.
  » Try full-body relaxation by starting at your head or feet and relaxing each part of the body, moving in a consistent direction.
- Alcohol sedates but is also a significant inhibitor of quality sleep.[194] Typically, the more alcohol consumed closer to bedtime, the less restful sleep will be.
  » Consider setting an alcohol limit and cutoff time (e.g., one drink, four hours before bedtime).

- » Keep track of alcohol consumption and sleep quality to determine whether or not your consumption pattern is affecting your sleep.
- Tetrahydrocannabinol (THC), like alcohol, may help induce sleep but will significantly diminish the quality of sleep.
- Prescription sleep aids do not improve quality sleep. Sedation is not sleep, and sleep aids should be a last resort for improving sleep. This topic is covered more in the Prescription Medication chapter.
- Melatonin, as a supplement, may be beneficial. Studies show two main populations where taking melatonin helps: older people and those who are jet-lagged. Older people do not produce as much melatonin and they release it earlier in the night, so taking a melatonin supplement can help improve their sleep. *Note: Even though research doesn't show melatonin to be particularly helpful for other populations, if you're getting a benefit from melatonin supplementation from a reputable manufacturer, you should not necessarily stop taking it.*[195] Bodies are unique, and the placebo effect can be substantial and real.

While Sleeping
- Strive for a whole night of sleep without wake-ups by using the bathroom before bed, limiting the amount of water before bed that will result in you waking up, and reducing or eliminating the aforementioned influences.
- Lower your bedroom temperature to 65 to 68 degrees Fahrenheit. Your core body temperature needs to drop by 2 to 3 degrees to initiate sleep. If your feet, hands, or skin are cold, warm them up with socks, gloves, a warm water bottle in your bed, or a hot shower. It may seem counterintuitive, but warmer extremities and skin provide more blood flow, making it easier for the body to drop the core temperature by radiating heat away.
- Consider removing clocks from the bedroom. Staring at a clock and watching time pass increases anxiety for some and reduces the

chance of falling asleep. Clocks that emit light may also disrupt sleep.
- Create an associative environment for sleep in your bed and bedroom:
  » Don't lie in bed awake for too long; your body will start to associate the bed with wakefulness and anxiety. If you have problems falling asleep, get up and do a relaxing activity such as reading or meditating. When you start to feel tired, go back to bed.
  » The bed/bedroom is best used for sleeping and sex. Refrain from working in the bed/bedroom, watching hours of TV in bed, or exercising in the bedroom because the brain associates the area with those activities instead of sleep.
- Consider sleeping separately from your partner. Disruptions from a partner can be one of the major causes of low-quality sleep, so sleeping apart might benefit both of you. Better sleep results in a better mood, better interpersonal relationships, and better sex hormones and desire.
- Do not fall asleep with the radio or TV on or while listening to a podcast. The brain continues to process the audio while we are sleeping.

Conclusion

Breathing and sleeping are critical activities for life, and maintaining and optimizing both over a lifetime will lead to better brain and overall health. Problems in these areas can have negative consequences as soon as the next day and can compound over a lifetime. Understanding these possible issues will lead to earlier interventions. There are strategies that help to identify and improve sleep and breathing issues that keep us from feeling our best and performing well. As with other recommendations in this book, it is advisable not to try to change everything at once and to seek out experts for their help when needed.

6

Prolonged Stress

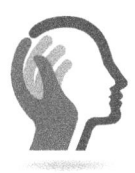

STRESS IS A PROTECTIVE REACTION by the body that has kept humans alive for centuries. When we were exposed to predators or faced dwindling food supplies, for example, our "fight-or-flight" response switched on and spurred us to action. Modern society has added many new stressors that activate the same stress response: constant social and technological connectedness, professional demands, societal demands, persistent crises (political, economic, environmental, or health), and the lure of social media, among others.

Stress has become such an accepted aspect of our lives that we often discount its effects and the toll it takes on the body. Although stress can be a natural, beneficial part of life that moves us to take on new challenges and increases our capabilities, it is most commonly experienced as something closer to "distress," which is the type of stress we discuss here.

This chapter discusses the ways in which the body reacts to stress, the physical and emotional symptoms of stress, how cortisol and other hormones contribute to diagnoses of Alzheimer's and other forms of dementia, and approaches for managing stress and the stress response.

The Impact of Stress on the Brain

Our bodies are designed to handle brief episodes of stress. In the face of a perceived threat, the body's built-in stress response activates the sympathetic nervous system. The heart beats faster than normal, blood pressure rises, and muscles tighten. Once the perceived threat passes, stress hormones normalize and heart rate slows, allowing the body to relax and go back into a parasympathetic or "rest-and-digest" state. People experience stress at all ages, and research shows that our memories are not as effective in times of stress. Even college students who experience stress have a harder time recalling information.[196]

Research tells us that as the brain ages, it has a harder time dealing with stress.[197] A 35-year longitudinal study showed that individuals, particularly women, who experienced psychological stress in midlife were at far greater risk of developing Alzheimer's dementia.[198] In the presence of stress, cell glucocorticoid receptors don't function as well, thereby releasing free (toxic) cortisol that can damage the brain.

As our world has become more stressful due to electronic devices, social media, the amount of information we're exposed to from multiple sources, and myriad other factors, people may feel fearful, anxious, and overwhelmed, and these feelings may be persistent and unrelenting. The sympathetic nervous system, in response, remains engaged and on alert, which makes relaxation nearly impossible. For many people, sleep, digestion, and the cardiovascular system are impacted.[199] During even a short period of time, being in a sympathetic state can take a significant toll on the body and the brain.

Continuous stress induces a chronic fear state in the brain. This fear activates the body's most primal "fight or flight" response (or "freeze" in potentially life-threatening situations). Different regions of the brain then react. The brain's emotional center, called the amygdala, sends a distress signal to the hypothalamus. The hypothalamus then sends signals to the rest of the body to react to the distress through the sympathetic nervous system, raising the heart rate and sending adrenaline to the body. This activation of the most primitive "reptilian" brain — the part that controls our involuntary functions — shuts down a critically important region of the brain called the prefrontal cortex. The immune system also becomes involved, releasing cytokines that lead to brain inflammation.[200] Cytokines are chemical messengers that signal immune cells to fight pathogens and other harmful substances.

One of the jobs of the prefrontal cortex is to send comforting messages to the brain's amygdala and insula. The amygdala controls emotions and specific aspects of memory function, while the insula soothes traumatic experiences. When the prefrontal area (our executive function control center) shuts down from continual stress, anxiety and tension may take over, and healthier emotions such as compassion and empathy are suppressed. This, in turn, may cause one to react to life in negative ways. All of this makes it difficult to be happy, joyful, loving, and fulfilled as a human being. Being in a sympathetic state can cause feelings of sadness and depression and the potential for cognitive decline.[201] The goal is to counter and prevent the chronic stress response and activate the parasympathetic nervous system, which allows us to rest and digest.

Cortisol

How does cognitive impairment develop from these stressful experiences? Stress elevates a hormone called cortisol which performs a wide variety of functions in the body, from regulating blood sugar and hormones to creating the fight-or-flight response in times of stress. Animal studies have shown that excessive secretion of corticosteroids raises deposits of beta amyloid plaques and fibrillary tangles.[202, 203] Amyloid beta and tau proteins are two hallmarks of AD, and these accumulations cause the widespread loss of synaptic and neuronal function that underlies memory loss.[204, 205] There is a strong connection between stress and Alzheimer's and other forms of dementia, with studies showing that compared to healthy people, patients with Alzheimer's disease have elevated cortisol levels that appear early on in the disease progression and correlate with their degree of memory impairment.[206]

When cortisol crosses the blood-brain barrier in sufficient quantities, it can impede learning and memory by binding to brain receptors on neurons in specific areas such as the hippocampus (a primary memory center), the amygdala, and the frontal lobes.[207] Researchers have observed that individuals with hippocampal atrophy and cognitive decline have high cortisol concentrations and inflammatory cytokines such as interleukin-6 (IL-6). Research also indicates that chronic stress arousal activates multiple other inflammatory mediators, creating widespread inflammation in the brain, especially in the hippocampus. This massive flood of central inflammation is a hallmark of AD.[208, 209]

Identifying Stress and Stressors

A critical step in reducing the harmful effects of stress is to identify the causes and the degree to which stress is impacting the individual.

Numerous types of situations and events in our lives — even happy ones — can cause stress, including:
- Illness or injury
- Loss of a job
- Worries about money
- Divorce
- Death of a spouse, family member, and friends
- Difficult relationships with family or friends
- Getting married/remarried
- Moving to a new house
- Experiencing discrimination

There are populations that may be at greater risk for memory loss and dementia. Women and people of color may be especially affected due to societal prejudices and caregiving responsibilities, and these two groups make up a disproportionate share of Alzheimer's patients in the United States.[210, 211] Transgender and non-binary individuals (TNB) report higher subjective cognitive impairment, dementia diagnoses, and chronic conditions that compound dementia risk.[212] Higher levels of discrimination and marginalization lead to poorer mental health outcomes that also impact physical health throughout one's life.[213]

Stress may not appear to be triggered in response to an external event at the time it occurs; the effects may be delayed for some period of time. Researchers at Ohio University showed that ruminating on a long-past stressful incident can increase C-reactive protein levels, a marker of inflammation in the body. The Ohio study — the first of its kind to directly measure this effect — has broad implications throughout the medical world since inflammation is a hallmark of most diseases, from diabetes to heart disease, cancer, and Alzheimer's.[214]

A great deal of stress is generated by thought and emotional patterns that may appear to be triggered by external events but are more related to an internally generated set of beliefs, expectations, and attitudes toward life, oneself, or others.[215] Predispositions are perspectives through which a person can look at any situation or trigger and find evidence that their beliefs are accurate. Examples: "I always get the short end of the stick." "No matter how hard I try, nothing works for me." "I'm just stupid." "It runs in the family." "I can't trust anyone."

Underneath these theme statements lie unresolved emotional issues and traumatic histories. Such habits of negative thinking and speaking incline people to move toward situations characterized by pain, hopelessness, and stress rather than those that offer more optimistic, peaceful possibilities. Psychotherapy, including cognitive behavioral therapy (CBT) or dialectical behavior therapy (DBT), can often help address these stress-producing patterns. However, several studies have shown that the effectiveness of the therapeutic experience depends less on the type of therapy chosen than on the quality — empathy, intuition, and experience — of the particular therapist.[216]

Physical and Emotional Stress
Severe emotional and physical trauma creates increased acute short-term stress and chronic long-term stress and unleashes inflammatory mediators. (The relationship between stress and inflammation is discussed in detail in the Physical and Emotional Trauma chapter.) It is not only isolated episodes of stress that lead to brain damage.[217] AD and other forms of emotional and cognitive dysfunction are also a function of the sum of cortisol exposure over a lifetime (especially in middle age and beyond).[218, 219, 220]

Technology
Technology has introduced many new benefits to modern life, but it has also come with some dynamics that the brain is not well equipped to handle. Social media is designed to maximize the amount of attention that we spend on each app or website, and one of the side effects can be anxiety and stress. Additionally, constant connectedness to work, or even friends and family, can create anxiety. Identifying which platforms and habits are having adverse effects can be a crucial step to reducing the stress in someone's life.

Signs and Symptoms of Stress
Stress is expressed differently by different people, which can make it difficult to identify.[221] Among the more familiar signs are physical symptoms, including:
- Gastrointestinal problems
- Headaches

- Muscle pain and tension
- Rapid heartbeat
- Teeth grinding
- Frequent colds or infection

Stress affects us emotionally as well. These less obvious symptoms are also warning signs:

- **Denial**: Having difficulty acknowledging stress and the effect it may have on one's self and family
- **Anger/frustration**: Frequently feeling angry with others due to not feeling understood
- **Social withdrawal**: Withdrawing from friends, family, and favorite activities
- **Anxiety**: Feeling worried, nervous, or uneasy, typically about an imminent event or something with an uncertain outcome
- **Depression**: Feelings of severe despondency and dejection
- **Exhaustion**: Being so exhausted that completing necessary daily tasks is almost impossible
- **Sleep disorders**: Losing sleep frequently or having difficulty waking up
- **Irritability**: Acting moodier than usual and being subject to frequent outbursts of frustration or anger
- **Lack of concentration**: Inability to stay focused on tasks or conversations with others

Cognitive problems are among the most serious consequences of stress. There is compelling evidence linking an increased risk of AD in people reporting the following sources of stress:

- Experiencing higher levels of work-related stress[222]
- Having stress-prone personalities[223]
- Enduring early childhood stressors such as abuse, trauma, and neglect[224]
- Suffering from midlife stressors such as divorce, widowhood,

serious problems with children, or a spouse's alcohol abuse. In a study specific to women, the risk of later developing AD increased 20 percent for each additional stressor reported.[225]

Managing Stress and Its Impact

Everyone's experience of what causes stress or what they define as a "stressful situation" is different and will depend on past experiences and how comfortable someone is in a particular situation. When dealing with the stress in our lives, we need to be aware of our own stress triggers and how we personally view these situations. The considerations below are about creating a structure for a lower-stress life, followed by activities or practices that we might incorporate into our daily lives.

Ways to Reframe and Remove Stress

- Identify sources of stress in one's life and particular triggers. What are they, and when do they occur? An introvert may need some time alone every day.
- Remove oneself from or reduce exposure to these situations whenever possible.
- For situations that can't be avoided (such as family events), identify what might help to ease the situation.
- Play with different ways of interpreting a situation. For example, some elements may be beyond our control, and learning to accept these can reduce stress. However, we may be able to make changes to other elements that will reduce or eliminate some of the stress.
- Define and maintain boundaries that specify what behavior is and is not personally acceptable. Inform others of these new limits. This will help reduce feelings of obligation and make it easier to say no without feeling angry or guilty.
- Learn what environments/methods of relaxation help with transitions and lower stress.

- Remember, two heads are usually better than one, so reach out to someone. Share feelings with a trusted family member or friend — someone who will listen without judging or criticizing. If this is not possible, then seek out a good therapist.
- Change the environment. For example, if high levels of stimulation in an environment are causing stress, find a quiet place to relax and regroup.
- Get plenty of rest to help maintain and conserve energy.
- Take a break. If something becomes too difficult or frustrating, put it aside and come back to it later. Some people have found positive affirmations, mantras, or expressions of faith to be especially helpful.

Ways to Manage Stress and Create Resilience

Stress can be reduced through physical, mental, and emotional channels. Each individual will find what is personally nurturing and enjoyable and what is most helpful in restoring a clear mind and relaxed body. For example:

- Exercise
- Eat a healthy diet
- Get plenty of sleep
- Go for a walk or hike outside
- Enjoy the unconditional love of a pet
- Journal about thoughts and feelings
- Take a long bath
- Spend time gardening
- Listen to music
- Watch a television program or read a book you find enjoyable
- Stay connected to supportive family and friends
- Take regular breaks from the news
- Regularly step away from your computer and smartphone, especially in the evening
- Get a massage

- Practice yoga
- Do some deep breathing exercises
- Meditate

It may be easy to initiate some of the activities, and others may feel more difficult, especially if one has been experiencing a prolonged period of stress. A health and wellness coach, life coach, or therapist can be helpful in identifying relaxing types of activities, setting goals, and gently holding clients accountable.

Mindfulness and Meditation

One of the best methods for mental fitness and stress management is mindfulness and meditation. The mental health and stress-relieving benefits of cultivating a mindfulness or meditation practice are well documented,[226, 227] and their benefits are directly linked to the reduction of cognitive decline.

Numerous studies have demonstrated that meditation reduces stress and cortisol levels and improves multiple health and cognition measures.[228] For example, one research team launched a preliminary investigation to determine if putting subjects with memory loss through a simple eight-week meditation program could improve memory and cerebral blood flow (CBF). After meditation training, participant scores on neuropsychological tests of verbal fluency and logical memory were significantly enhanced, and so was cerebral blood flow.[229] In another study, ten participants were asked to meditate for 11 minutes twice daily for eight weeks. Before and after the intervention, participants were measured for perceived stress, sleep, mood, memory functioning, and blood pressure. Participants demonstrated improvement in all major outcomes.[230]

There are countless meditation techniques that provide health benefits. The focus in the next section is on a technique called Kirtan Kriya, a chanting meditation exercise which is easy for individuals of all ages to learn and practice and which also has a positive impact on memory.

Kirtan Kriya (KK)

Kirtan Kriya (pronounced KEER-tun KREE-a) is a type of meditation from the Kundalini yoga tradition, and it has been practiced for thousands of years. Close to two decades of medical research on KK have demonstrated compelling positive results when it comes to memory loss. In one study where 75 percent of the subjects were women (a population especially vulnerable to AD), there was a highly significant finding: KK reversed memory loss and helped create enhanced psychological and spiritual well-being.[231]

In another study of caregivers and their patients — people with subjective cognitive decline or mild cognitive impairment and both at high risk for developing AD — KK was successfully employed to improve memory in both groups.[232, 233] Kirtan Kriya has also been shown to improve sleep, decrease depression, reduce anxiety, down-regulate inflammatory genes, up-regulate immune system genes, improve insulin and glucose regulatory genes, and increase telomerase, an enzyme that helps to protect our DNA from damage and aging, by 43 percent. Kirtan Kriya also improves psychological well-being and spiritual connection, factors that help to maintain cognitive function and prevent AD.[234, 235]

Kirtan Kriya is sometimes called a singing exercise, as it involves singing the sounds "Sa Ta Na Ma" and using repetitive finger movements, or mudras. This nonreligious practice can be adapted to several lengths, but practicing it for just 12 minutes a day has been shown to reduce stress levels, improve cognition, and increase activity in areas of the brain central to memory.[236] This practice also causes positive biochemical changes in the brain. Research has revealed that coordinating the fingertip position with the sounds enhances blood flow within the brain's motor sensory area.[237]

Each component of Kirtan Kriya calls on a specific part of the neurological system, and each is vital to the whole to reap the full benefit of the practice. Replacing the Kirtan Kriya sounds with other sounds, engaging in different types of meditations, or performing other relaxing tasks have not been proven to be as effective. The Alzheimer's Research and Prevention Foundation recommends practicing the traditional Kirtan Kriya daily as described below to experience a clearer mind and maintain the benefits of the exercise.[238]

How Do You Practice Kirtan Kriya?
Practicing the Kirtan Kriya engages us physically and mentally, which is why it is so effective:
- Sit with your spine straight.
- Close your eyes.
- Repeat the "Sa Ta Na Ma" sounds (or mantra).
- Simultaneously, use the mudras or KK finger positions:
  » On Sa, touch the index fingers of each hand to your thumbs.
  » On Ta, touch your middle fingers to your thumbs.
  » On Na, touch your ring fingers to your thumbs.
  » On Ma, touch your little fingers to your thumbs.
- Vary the way you express the sounds:
  » For two minutes, sing in your normal voice.
  » For the next two minutes, sing in a whisper.
  » For the next four minutes, say the sounds silently to yourself.
  » Then reverse the order, whispering for two minutes, and then speaking out loud for two minutes.
  » The practice takes a total of 12 minutes.
- With each syllable, imagine the sound flowing down through the top of your head and out the middle of your forehead (your third eye point), focusing your attention on this L shape. Keep your eyes closed and chant in a continuous flow.

Where to Find Meditations and the Kirtan Kriya
There is an endless number of good meditation resources available due to a surge in its popularity. If you have found a good resource

that works for you, that is likely your best option. An example and suggested melody for an 11-minute version of the Kirtan Kriya can be found at https://youtu.be/jfKEAiwrgeY. Another free resource called Insight Timer has thousands of free meditations and teachings from excellent practitioners and is one of the best timers for those who prefer unguided meditation. There are good examples of guided Kirtan Kriya there as well.

Conclusion

While stress may seem to be ever present in our busy, fast-paced lives, unremitting stress without periods of relaxation have profound effects on the brain. Prolonged stress also has been shown to affect overall and long-term health and well-being. Meditation in general, and Kirtan Kriya specifically, along with other strategies discussed in this section, may be beneficial in reducing stress, are important for regular self-care, and are part of an integrated AD prevention program.

PART TWO

THE DEEPER DIVE

AS WE HAVE SEEN IN THE PREVIOUS CHAPTERS, each of us has the opportunity to safeguard our health by paying attention to our habits and lifestyle practices. Maintaining a healthy lifestyle goes a long way toward ensuring that the brain is functioning optimally. We live in a complex world, however, that is changing rapidly due to external factors that impact our bodies, our brains, and our genes. In this section, we will discuss less obvious factors that influence brain health and require intervention of some kind; this typically includes testing and treatment under the care of a specially trained professional.

Issues such as Lyme disease; mold, heavy metals, and other toxicities; hormonal imbalances; infections that cause inflammation; and untreated emotional and physical trauma may not be immediately associated with brain health but are now known to potentially cause dementia. Some of these problematic conditions have been identified and understood only in the past 40 years due to research and broader understanding of these issues. It has taken a similarly long time to develop appropriate treatments, whether addressing mold toxicity or determining a safe and effective protocol to administer bioidentical hormone replacement.

Being aware of the many factors that impact brain health is critical because, in most cases, the body suffers insults from multiple sources. In some cases, these insults do not produce noticeable symptoms. Looking at the body and brain as an integrative whole is a first step in identifying what combination of factors may be contributing to cognitive problems and, therefore, which diagnostic tests are appropriate. In many cases, individuals are able to identify the most likely factors contributing to their memory issues, and recounting their history to an experienced integrative, holistic, or naturopathic practitioner can point toward an initial course of testing and treatment.

The following chapters discuss hormonal imbalances, sources and effects of toxins and heavy metals, infections and pathogens that cause inflammation in the body and the brain, prescription medications, and physical and emotional trauma. These causes of memory loss often take longer to treat due to their complexity, testing that may be required, the need to identify qualified practitioners, and understanding that varied approaches may be necessary. For that reason, it is recommended that any memory issue be addressed as early as possible because early intervention increases the likelihood of successful outcomes in treating and restoring cognitive health.

7

Hormones

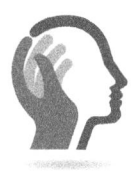

HORMONES ARE, BY DEFINITION, MESSAGING MOLECULES made in glands in one part of the body and then transported by the circulatory system to cells throughout the body. The messages that hormones bring to the cells affect our body's processes, from bone strength to our brains' health and optimal functioning. All of our basic metabolic processes, including digestion, heart function, respiration, kidney function, detoxification, sleep, and tissue repair depend on our hormonal messaging system. When our hormones are in balance, we feel well and have a better quality of life.

Hormones come in a few different forms. Some hormones, such as norepinephrine or noradrenaline, help during physically, mentally, and emotionally stressful times. Other hormones, like insulin, are derived from amino acids resulting from protein metabolism. Other hormones are derived from cholesterol; these are the sex steroid hormones. Male and female sex hormones and all other hormones circulate via the bloodstream to cells throughout the body.

There is growing evidence linking disruptions in the endocrine system to the pathogenesis of AD and other dementias. In multiple studies, the development of dementia has been linked to abnormal functioning of critical hormones in the following ways:

- Low production of thyroid hormones[239]
- Low estrogen production[240]
- Low testosterone production[241]
- An imbalance of progesterone and estrogen[242]
- Changes in cholesterol[243]
- Insulin resistance[244]
- Elevated cortisol[245]

Thyroid and Brain Function

Thyroid hormone functions as the growth, development, and repair hormone. The thyroid gland in front of the neck controls metabolic function in every cell of the body through the thyroid hormones T4 and T3. T3 is integral to hundreds of physiological processes, including bone metabolism, gastrointestinal function and acid production, regulation of growth hormone, insulin and glucose metabolism, protein synthesis, and brain chemistry regulation.

The brain is saturated with thyroid receptors, and healthy thyroid function is essential for healthy brain function. Conversely, a healthy brain and adequate production of serotonin and dopamine are necessary for healthy thyroid function. Through a series of biochemical steps, tyrosine, an amino acid derived from protein, is eventually converted into T4 and T3 by addition of iodine molecules. The active form of thyroid hormone, T3, turns on or slows down metabolic function and is therefore responsible for much of our thyroid's healthy functioning. The liver, gastrointestinal tract, heart, muscle, and nerves all play a role in converting most of the T4 in our bodies into T3. Our body relies on specific vitamins, nutrients, and other hormones to make this process work.

The brain can become impaired (sometimes severely) if the body is not making enough of the thyroid hormone's active form (T3). Untreated hypothyroidism, or an underactive thyroid gland, can lead to a host of other health problems, including depression and dementia.[246]

The most common symptoms of hypothyroidism can be seen in the following:

Symptoms of Hypothyroidism	
Common Symptoms	
• Brain fog • Cold body, hands, and feet • Constipation • Depression • Dementia	• Dry skin • Hair loss • Low body temperature • Low energy, fatigue • Puffiness in face
Additional Symptoms	
• Diminished libido • Feeling nervous and emotional • Heavy, irregular periods • Hoarseness • Insomnia (or needing excessive sleep)	• Joint and muscle pain, stiffness, swelling • Muscle weakness • Slow digestion • Slowed heart rate • Weight gain

How Hashimoto's Thyroiditis Develops

Twenty-seven million Americans are affected by thyroid malfunction, the most common form being Hashimoto's thyroiditis. In Hashimoto's, the body makes antibodies in response to inflammatory trigger foods (sugar, wheat, dairy), infections, and toxins, which can permeate the intestinal lining.[247] It may be that some antibodies mistake thyroid tissue for a foreign invader and attack it. Initially, Hashimoto's remains silent, and the thyroid functions normally. As thyroid damage continues, hormone release is inconsistent, and individuals may experience the effects of having too much or too little hormone in circulation. Eventually, thyroid function will stop completely, and classic hypothyroidism occurs.

Diagnosing Thyroid Problems
A blood test will identify signs of Hashimoto's, which are thyroid peroxidase (anti-TPO) and thyroglobulin (anti-Tgb) antibodies. These antibodies are generally created by the combination of an environmental stressor and bacterial imbalance in the gut leading to "leaky gut" (more information can be found in the Food Sensitivities section of the chapter on Inflammation and Infections). If found early, it is possible to reverse this autoimmune disease by removing problematic foods, infections and toxins, and healing the gut. Individuals with Hashimoto's are at an increased risk of developing other autoimmune conditions; therefore, addressing the immune response's root cause(s) is critically important. Unfortunately, Hashimoto's often progresses unrecognized, leading to irreversible damage to the thyroid. At that point, thyroid hormone replacement is usually necessary. One way to determine whether you have an underactive thyroid is to take your temperature upon waking and one or two other times throughout the day. A basal or early morning temperature below 97.8 degrees Fahrenheit (oral) may suggest low thyroid function.

Tests to Request From Your Doctor
Many doctors focus attention almost exclusively on T4, the inactive form of thyroid hormone. If you have symptoms of hypothyroidism or an underactive metabolism, your doctor should check for thyroid peroxidase and thyroglobulin antibodies, free and total T4 (thyroxine), free and total T3 (triiodothyronine), reverse T3 (rT3), and thyroid-stimulating hormone (TSH).

Healing Your Thyroid
If tests show evidence of autoimmune thyroiditis or low hormone levels, following these steps (with the help of an integrative/functional medicine practitioner) can restore thyroid balance:

- Improve your nutrition by getting amino acids from proteins, essential vitamins (including B vitamins and vitamins C and D), and minerals (such as selenium, iron, iodine, and zinc).
- Avoid inflammatory foods, including gluten and dairy. Grains and legumes may also need to be eliminated. Build a healthy gut by addressing infections, parasites, and food allergens (through testing and treatment), and discuss reducing or eliminating acid-blocking medications with your doctor.
- Because the thyroid and the adrenal glands supply and deliver hormones throughout the body, it is important to make sure the adrenals are functioning well. Your doctor will work with you to optimize cortisol levels by suggesting many of the steps mentioned here, such as lowering stress and sugar in the diet.
- Reduce your body's toxic burden: Avoid exposure to toxins and support your body's detoxification mechanisms. See the chapter on Toxins for more information.
- Heal any lingering infections. If you feel inflammation or pain in the body and the cause has not been identified, seek help to find out why and address it. Infections that go undetected are common and may be in the mouth or other areas of the body that have recently experienced invasive procedures. Another cause of infections are insect and tick bites and mold exposure.
- Relieve stress through regular activities such as yoga, meditation, prayer, and paced breathing.
- Make rest a priority by getting 7 to 8 hours of solid sleep nightly.
- Move your body every day by doing some form of exercise.

Sex Hormones

Effects on the Body and Brain Health
The sex steroid hormones discussed here include estrogens, progesterone, and testosterone. These hormones support healthy mood and

behavior by their regulation of brain neurotransmitters. Estrogen activates serotonin (the happy-sad neurotransmitter) receptors in both men and women and increases dopamine (the focusing and commitment neurotransmitter) receptors in women. Progesterone supports gamma-aminobutyric acid or GABA (the relaxing neurotransmitter) receptors in both men and women. Testosterone increases dopamine receptors in men. Acetylcholine (the thinking neurotransmitter) receptors are activated in women by estrogens and in men by testosterone.

As we age, our hormone levels decrease. Symptoms of lower hormone levels include fatigue, graying and loss of hair, decreased muscle tone and strength, joint aches and pains, thinning of bones, and sagging skin. Women may have weak bladder and vaginal dryness issues, while men experience erectile dysfunction and prostate problems. Newly menopausal women may feel depressed, sedentary, and lack motivation, all of which speaks to the strong connection between aging, lower hormone levels, and optimal health. In the brain, lower sex hormones may contribute to increased inflammation, lower oxygenation, and diminished function of the neurotransmitters.[248] The following sections provide a brief description of each hormone's role in the body, followed by the relationship of the sex hormones in maintaining brain health.

Estrogens
Estrogens estradiol (E2), estrone (E1), and estriol (E3) are the primary female sex steroid hormones. They promote the health of the reproductive system and female fertility in women. The organs most affected include breast tissue, the uterus, and ovaries. Estrogens in both men and women also promote the health of the heart, bones, liver, and brain. In bones, estrogens prevent excessive bone breakdown. Estradiol is the strongest of the trio, and estriol the weakest. Estrone is a moderately strong estrogen, but it can be problematic if levels are too high in both men and women because it is created by the activation of an enzyme called aromatase, caused by inflammation.[249]

Testosterone

Testosterone performs a similar function in men as estrogen does in women. Optimal functioning of the male reproductive system and male fertility depends on healthy levels of testosterone. In both men and women, testosterone plays a role in sexual energy and libido. Testosterone in men is the hormone responsible for muscle growth and repair and it also supports building strong bones.

Sexual energy or libido suffers in both men and women when testosterone is low. Lack of focus and commitment can be a sign of low testosterone in either sex. Mentally, people struggle to remember things that were easy to recall before. Weight training is an excellent way to build back testosterone in both men and women; weight training and other ways of building lean muscle mass have been shown in 60- to 75-year-olds to reverse the biological clock ten years after a six-month training program.[250]

Progesterone

Progesterone in women is the balancing hormone to estrogens. Wherever there are estrogen receptors in the body, there are also progesterone receptors. These receptors are protein-created doorways into the cells that the hormones access for entry. Together, estrogens and progesterone regulate the menstrual cycle and help support female fertility. Progesterone also has positive effects as a natural diuretic helping the kidneys to filter urine. Along with estrogens and testosterone, progesterone positively impacts the heart, blood vessels, bone, and brain. Wherever there are receptor sites for these hormones is where these hormones do their job supporting health and quality of life.

How to Support Brain Health

Estrogen, progesterone, and testosterone are called neurosteroids because they are also made in the brain and reduce brain inflammation. Studies show that estrogens started early in menopause (before age 60) help prevent cognitive decline in later years.[251] The positive benefits are not seen to the same degree in studies done on women starting estrogens after age 60. Transdermal hormones (applied topically or through a skin patch) are associated with positive cognitive outcomes for women with Alzheimer's disease.[252] Another study showed the long-term use of topical estradiol gel and oral micronized progesterone may reduce cognitive decline in postmenopausal women with mild cognitive impairment.[253] Hormones should be considered on a case-by-case basis and only with a doctor's guidance.

All three sex steroids have been shown to reduce brain inflammation. One mechanism may be the balancing and support to the brain's white blood cell system called microglia. When microglial cells are out of balance, there is increased brain inflammation. Estrogen, progesterone, and testosterone have been shown to support healthy microglia in the brain.[254, 255] Another reason for brain inflammation and associated cognitive decline is reduced oxygenation of the brain. This is seen in sleep apnea patients, as discussed in the Sleep and Breathing chapter. Studies show that testosterone can protect the brain from neuronal damage due to reduced oxygenation of neuronal cells.[256] Testosterone has also been shown to be neuroprotective after traumatic brain injury.[257]

Many of the possible reasons for memory loss, cognitive decline, and dementia involve reduced oxygen levels (hypoxia) in the brain and chronic inflammation. It would make sense to support healthy sex steroid hormone levels because they are neuroprotective in the face of any hypoxic or inflammatory stress on the brain.[258] Testosterone has been shown in men and women to protect against neurodegeneration that results from the buildup of beta amyloid protein in the hippocampus, the brain's major memory center.[259]

What to Do to Improve Hormone Levels and Brain Health
The use of bioidentical hormones can be helpful in preserving brain health as we age. The body already has the pathways and mecha-

nisms to utilize the bioidentical hormones in a way similar to our natural hormones. Physicians who are experienced with hormones can prescribe and/or have bioidentical hormones compounded for the individual patient. Anyone using these hormones needs to be monitored carefully to make sure that the hormones are in balance and that there are no unwanted effects.

Cholesterol and Lipids

Cholesterol, lipids, and their relationship to cognitive health is a complex subject with inconclusive research and different schools of thought. The amounts of high-density lipoprotein (HDL) cholesterol, known as "good cholesterol," and low-density lipoprotein (LDL) cholesterol, or "bad cholesterol," in the blood, as well as their ratio, are measures of the health of the cardiovascular system and thus the brain.

The brain contains approximately 20 percent of the body's cholesterol, and this waxy substance plays many roles. Cholesterol supports the health of cell membranes, allowing proper signaling and the transport of substances in and out of the cell. Cholesterol is also part of the makeup of vitamin D and many other hormones in the body, including estrogen and testosterone, so it makes sense to monitor and manage cholesterol levels for two main reasons:

- Heart health: High blood cholesterol is a modifiable cardiovascular risk factor, and cardiovascular disease is a key risk factor for cognitive decline and Alzheimer's disease.[260] For this reason, monitoring and managing blood cholesterol will likely have a positive effect on overall brain health.
- Brain health: Both abnormally high and low cholesterol show some relationship to cognitive decline:
  » Low HDL cholesterol: It may be surprising to hear that low cholesterol can be a problem because the emphasis is usually on lowering cholesterol levels. However, low HDL cholesterol in late life has been shown to be correlated with brain atrophy in

several brain structures.[261, 262] One recommendation stemming from these findings is to keep total cholesterol above 150 while still maintaining an optimal LDL-P (low-density lipoprotein particles) level of 700 to 1,000.[263]

» High LDL cholesterol: A causal link between high levels of LDL-P and the development of cardiovascular disease (CVD) has been well documented. Elevated levels of LDL cholesterol are associated with increased risk of Alzheimer's,[264] while low levels (< 100 mg/dL) are correlated with slower cognitive decline as we age.[265]

Monitoring Cholesterol

If someone regularly visits their primary care physician, they are likely already monitoring their cholesterol levels through the standard lipid panel of blood tests (total cholesterol, LDL-C, HDL-C, triglycerides, lipid ratios).[266] There are more advanced tests that help provide a clearer picture of cardiovascular disease risk, such as the low-density lipoprotein particle test (LDL-P), which tests for the number of particles in the blood instead of the total mass.[267] There is genuine disagreement as to which metrics are most important for monitoring cardiovascular risk and dementia risk; the field of lipidology is far from settled science.

Other tests you may consider discussing with your doctor are oxidized LDL (sdLDL or oxLDL), lipid subparticles (ApoA, ApoB, Lp(a), LPIR), homocysteine, inflammatory markers (hs-CRP), insulin resistance (HbA1c, fasting insulin), and a calcium score or rapid calcium CT scan of the heart. This test can quantify the amount of calcium in the coronary blood vessels. The higher the level of calcium, the more inflammation in the blood vessels. This is the body's way of dealing with inflammation: Calcium is deposited in the inflamed area, almost like a patch or Band-Aid. Cholesterol is then deposited on top of the calcium. White blood cells called foam cells also contribute to the "patch" that creates atherosclerosis in the blood vessels.[268]

Managing Cholesterol

The most substantial evidence suggests that managing cholesterol in midlife (ages 45 to 65) reduces Alzheimer's risk and protects against cognitive decline.[269] There is less evidence for the effects of managing high cholesterol in late-life. There have been some studies that suggest benefits of using statins as an AD treatment,[270] but statins have side effects and pose some risks. A discussion about statins, their uses, and side effects is in the Prescription Medication chapter.

There are two approaches to managing blood cholesterol levels: lifestyle changes (Mediterranean diet, exercise, and stress management) and medications. With each approach, there are many options, and generally, the recommendation is to try to lower cholesterol levels through lifestyle changes before using medications.

Lifestyle Tools

The three primary means of controlling cholesterol with lifestyle factors are reducing saturated fat in the diet, losing weight, and increasing exercise. The best methods for these are discussed in the Nutrition and Supplements and Physical Activity chapters. Additional strategies include reducing inflammation, optimizing hormones, reducing stress, and treating insulin resistance. Most research studies that show the positive effects on cognition when cholesterol is lowered in midlife used statins, not lifestyle changes. That said, the above lifestyle factors are common recommendations for lowering cholesterol and promoting brain health. Trying several lifestyle approaches may be necessary to determine which one works best for an individual.

Medications

The use of statins to control midlife cholesterol has been shown to reduce the risk of cognitive decline in late-life.[271, 272] The Prescription Medication chapter includes a discussion of statins and the cognitive and other potential risks of using these medications. In *Risk Reduction of Cognitive Decline and Dementia: WHO Guidelines*, the World Health Organization recommends the management of high cholesterol in midlife to reduce the risk of cognitive decline and dementia. They also state that, in their view, the benefit of treating high cholesterol outweighs the risks of statin drug use.

What About People with the ApoE4 Allele and Other Genes?
The cholesterol issue is amplified for people with one or two ApoE4 alleles, which reduces the body's cholesterol transport capability.[273] People with this gene typically are at higher risk for cardiovascular disease and Alzheimer's disease. The best approach is to work with a doctor familiar with ApoE4; additional resources can be found at ApoE4.info. The approach to cholesterol and lipid management should be highly individualized, taking into account genomics and other biomarkers. There are many other genes that affect the body's relationship with cholesterol and lipids.

Insulin

Insulin is the primary hormone responsible for regulating blood sugar — our main energy fuel — by stimulating absorption of glucose from the bloodstream into the cell. Made in the pancreas, it is released into the bloodstream in response to carbohydrate consumption.

When glucose metabolism is working normally, blood sugar goes up after a meal, insulin is released, and both glucose and insulin drop within a two-hour period. Consistently high blood sugar levels can lead to insulin resistance, when cells become insensitive to the actions of insulin. Frequent snacking and consuming highly processed carbs such as breads, pasta, white rice, and desserts all contribute to high blood sugar levels and insulin resistance. Over time, insulin resistance leads to impaired glucose metabolism, prediabetes, and eventually diabetes.

The process of linking high blood sugar to inflammation is called glycation, and it occurs when sugar binds to protein and fat, creating deformed molecules known as AGEs: advanced glycation end products. AGEs do not naturally form in the body when it is metabolically healthy, so when they are detected, it signals chronic inflammation. Inside the brain, this foreign sugar and protein combination is toxic and degenerative over time.[274]

Alzheimer's disease, sometimes referred to as Type 3 diabetes, may be the manifestation of chronically elevated blood sugar, insulin resistance, inflammation, and oxidative stress (internal "rusting"). Insulin on its own is not the cause of cognitive impairment; rather, it's the cellular resistance that develops as a result of chronically elevated blood sugar that leads to tissue damage related to cognitive impairment.

Conclusion

Maintaining optimal hormone levels is vital for proper brain function throughout life, and particularly as we age. In this chapter we addressed the relationship between brain health and the hormones insulin, cholesterol, estrogen, progesterone, testosterone, thyroid, and cortisol. Each hormone performs different functions in the body and requires specialized testing to determine whether they are at optimal levels. It is critical to understand how they all work together because keeping one's hormone levels balanced is an important step in building long-term cognitive and overall health. Sharp Again suggests that patients work with an endocrinologist or functional medicine doctor with hormone expertise to find the best solutions to their unique situation.

8
Toxins

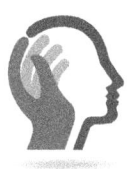

AS OUR WORLD HAS BECOME MORE fast paced, automated, and "processed," we are regularly exposed to chemicals, heavy metals, and other toxicants, which are the by-products of our way of life. The body will eliminate toxins if it can or store them in fat tissue. Repeated daily exposures to pollutants, over decades, often results in a "toxic body burden." Once this burden becomes too much for our bodies to manage, toxins may be deposited in our organs and we will begin to experience disease symptoms, including neuroinflammation and cognitive impairment.

What contributes to this "toxic body burden"? Everything from chemical-dependent industrial agriculture, forest, land, and water management; artificial food additives; and pollutants in our water and air to chemicals in our household cleaning products and furnishings. Our soil has been degraded of nutrients, and streams, rivers, and land have been polluted with toxic sewage from feedlots, pesticides and herbicides, and industrial operations. Over 86,000 chemicals are used in the United States, many in our food, homes, and personal care products. Very few have been effectively tested for impact on human health, and we are seeing numerous and serious effects on child and adult development. Some of these chemicals have been connected to autism,[275] asthma,[276] allergies,[277] learning difficulties,[278] reproductive issues,[279] Parkinson's,[280] and dementia.[281]

According to a diverse range of sources, from studies to experts on health, most people have accumulated toxic pollutants, including heavy metals, flame retardants, and pesticide residues within their bodies.[282, 283] It has been shown that many of these toxicants have neurodegenerative as well as neurodevelopmental impacts as a result of various mechanisms, including neuronal mitochondrial toxicity and disruption of neurotransmitter regulation.[284] Eliminating these toxicants from the body can help to diminish their adverse effects and restore normal physiological functions.

The ability to naturally rid the body of toxins varies from person to person. There are gene variants that impede detoxification, for example. Our methylation cycle facilitates many vital functions in the body, such as hormone metabolism, neurotransmitter production, organ health, and detoxification. It is estimated that 30 percent of the population has at least one genetic mutation often referred to as MTHFR (methylenetetrahydrofolate reductase) that may disrupt the elimination of toxins from the body. Approximately 25 percent of Hispanic Americans and 10 to 15 percent of Caucasian Americans have two copies of the mutation, which impedes the breakdown of homocysteine, a marker of many conditions, including cardiovascular disease and inflammation, that may contribute to dementia.[285]

As individuals, we need to be vigilant about our own health and safety because the priorities of government agencies such as the Environmental Protection Agency (EPA) and Food and Drug Administration (FDA) often shift. Over time, more chemicals and toxins are introduced into our food and our environment. In the future, daily detoxification protocols may well become part of our routine.

Sources and Effects of Toxic Exposure

Air

After an intravenous line into a vein, the second fastest route of substances into the body is through inhalation via the mouth and lungs. From there, the substances go directly into the bloodstream. We experience constant exposure to airborne pollutants in the outside air and in our homes and workplaces every day.

Depending on their characteristics, air toxicants can reach the brain through several pathways. The effects of air pollution on the brain can then manifest as neuroinflammation, oxidative stress, and neurodegeneration.[286] Both the physical characteristics of an air particle itself and toxic compounds adsorbed on the particle may be responsible for the damage. Time of exposure also plays a crucial role in the extent of the damage. The breadth, strength, and consistency of the preclinical and clinical evidence provides a compelling argument that air pollution, especially traffic-derived pollution, causes central nervous system damage, and thus we can conclude there is a clear link between air pollution and neurological diseases.[287] This exposure to particulate matter can begin in childhood and accumulate in the body over time.

In a 2017 study, researchers at the University of Toronto reported in *The Lancet* that among the 6.6 million people in the province of Ontario, those living within 50 meters of a major road — where levels of fine pollutants are often ten times higher than just 150 meters away — were 12 percent more likely to develop dementia than people living more than 200 meters away.[288]

Urban centers tend to have more concentrated air pollutants, but wherever there is industry, there is often waste output, even in rural areas. Typically, the greater the exposure to airborne contaminants, the higher the incidence of cognitive impairment and dementia.[289] In the Women's Health Initiative Memory Study (WHIMS) and experimental mouse models, those women who carried the ApoE4 allele showed even greater cognitive impairment caused by fine particulate matter exposure. The study found that "residing in places with fine [particulate matter] exceeding EPA standards increased the risks for global cognitive decline and all-cause dementia respectively by 81 and 92 percent, with stronger adverse effects in ApoE 4/4 carriers [from both parents]." In this study, increased cerebral amyloid beta production was observed as well as changes in the hippocampus.[290]

As the climate is changing, we must also be aware of the effects of wildfires on brain health. In a study of nine emission sources, agriculture, traffic, coal combustion, and wildfires resulted in the strongest associations with dementia.[291]

The effects of nitrogen dioxide (NO2) in the respiratory system have been studied in children, where symptoms of exposure included irritation of the eyes, nose, and throat.[292] Nitrogen dioxide is produced when fossil fuels like coal, oil, methane gas, or diesel are burned at high temperatures. These sources include fuel used in cars, power plants, and off-road equipment. NO2 can also form indoors when fuels like wood or gas are burned. Researchers are most concerned with NO2's neurological impact; several studies have shown that a child's exposure to NO2 can result in ADHD and lower performance on neurobehavioral tests and overall cognitive function, verbal abilities, and executive functioning.[293, 294]

Unfortunately, the adverse effects of air pollution are seen in adults as well, especially those of advanced age. In Germany, China, and the United States, separate studies show that increases in air pollution were associated with difficulties in cognitive functioning and are thought to lead to dementia.[295]

Electromagnetic Frequencies

Electromagnetic frequency (EMF) is included in this chapter because it may directly harm the brain, thus increasing the risk of dementia. In addition, research studies have shown that EMFs affect the body more broadly in ways that can cumulatively add to the risk for dementia, including increased oxidative stress, sleep disturbances, psychological issues, and imbalances of the gut microbiome.

The easiest way to explain EMF is to begin by stating that the human body is a coherent, highly sensitive electrical system called the biofield, described as "the field of energy and information that surrounds and interpenetrates the human body."[296] Humans have evolved to live in a world that has native electrical frequency: a magnetic and electrical field from the earth and the sun that nurtures us and has kept us thriving. We have evolved with that natural frequency (Schumann Resonance), which vibrates at 7.83 Hz (or cycles) per second and surrounds and protects all living things on the planet.

Non-native electromagnetic fields are man-made and include microwave radiation, radio frequencies, and what is emitted from cell phones and towers, routers, and "smart" appliances — anything wireless. These are referred to as EMFs, and their frequencies may be disruptive for the human body.[297] EMFs have frequencies of up to 300 Hz. Radiofrequency electromagnetic fields (RF-EMFs) are produced through use of large-scale wireless equipment and data transmission. RF-EMF frequencies range from 3 kHz (or 3,000 Hz) to 300 GHz (or 300 billion Hz).

Symptoms and Risks of EMF Exposure
Because our exposure to more powerful frequencies is relatively new, research is ongoing. As far back as 1997, however, studies have shown a slight increased risk between EMF exposure and dementia.[298] A 2007 study showed that occupational EMF exposure increased the risk of developing Alzheimer's disease.[299] In 2015, almost 200 scientists in Europe signed an open letter[300] expressing concern about allowing 5G frequency to be rolled out around the globe.

The reported health effects of EMF exposure are wide-ranging and include achiness, fatigue, headaches, and insomnia. In a study on the effects of RF-EMF on the central nervous system, the authors noted that "significant statistical results have been reported by various epidemiological studies on cognitive disorders such as headache, tremor, dizziness, memory loss, loss of concentration, and sleep disturbance due to RF-EMF."[301] Other effects include elevated blood pressure and lipid levels.[302, 303]

With prolonged exposure to high levels of EMFs, research has shown debilitating psychological effects, including depression-like neurobehavioral disorders and gut microbiota imbalance.[304, 305] A 2018 study reported that chronic exposure to EMF fields is also a risk factor for poor sleep quality, stress, anxiety, and depression,[306] which may be contributing to a higher incidence of these conditions in the young adult population.

Fetuses can be exposed to EMFs from the earliest stages of development.[307, 308] Studies over the past two decades show that children exposed to high levels of EMFs in the womb experienced disruptions in brain development and sleep patterns and increased asthma, among other issues.[309]

Other Effects of EMFs

Smart TVs, electric clocks, cell phones, and iPads are sources of EMF exposure and are frequently placed in the bedroom. This exposure suppresses the production of melatonin, which causes sleep issues in both children and adults. In addition, these devices emit both blue light and LED light, which affects circadian rhythm and sleep.[310] As discussed in detail in the chapter on Sleep, quality sleep is necessary for memory consolidation and detoxification of the brain, and without it, we are at higher risk for dementia.

EMFs may also cause dehydration and harmful oxidative stress in the body.[311, 312] Dr. Martin Pall, professor emeritus of biochemistry and basic medical sciences at Washington State University, has researched the effects of EMFs on the human body. He states that EMFs stimulate the body's voltage-gated calcium channels, which are found in neurons and muscle cells. This activity increases intracellular calcium, which can then produce harmful levels of nitric oxide, potentially leading to dangerous free radicals circulating in the body.[313] Oxidative stress from free radicals has been linked to Alzheimer's and causes chronic diseases including cancer, diabetes, cardiovascular disease, autoimmune issues, and infertility. It also causes a breakdown of the blood-brain barrier, which is supposed to prevent toxins and pathogens in the circulatory system from entering the brain.[314]

One other body area affected by EMFs is the gut microbiome. Gut health is directly related to brain health, with a significant portion of the body's neurotransmitters being generated in the gut. Exposure to electromagnetic frequency has been shown to suppress beneficial microbes in the gut, disturbing the balance of the gut microbiome and resulting in an increase of pathogens. E. coli and listeria, for example, grow at a faster rate when exposed to electromagnetic frequencies.[315]

Researchers and practitioners in the field believe that exposure to Wi-Fi frequency and electronic devices exacerbates all other toxic exposures.[316] For example, exposure to heavy metals (like the mercury found in "silver" amalgam fillings) is known to be toxic. Frequent cell phone use can multiply the effect, liberating up to 600 times more amalgam and exposing the body to significantly more mercury.[317] EMFs are pervasive and getting stronger as technology companies have moved to the 5G wireless standard.

Food
We have evidence that specific foods can adversely impact cognitive function, and, conversely, foods that support the body and brain can enhance mental functioning. For example, a 2017 study of 317 Korean adolescents' consumption of noodles, fast food, and Coca-Cola showed a negative correlation on neurocognitive tests. Vitamins B1 and B6 and vitamin C, as well as mushrooms and nuts, showed a positive correlation.[318]

The following are foods or food substances that may be toxic to the brain.

- *Aspartame*

Like MSG (see next), there are studies citing the safety of aspartame and others showing harmful effects including headaches, dementia, and seizures.[319] Aspartame is a sugar substitute found in beverages, toothpaste, and other food products; it is also in many medications. A 2017 review of the literature found that aspartame may be responsible for adverse neurobehavioral health outcomes.[320] In another study, while aspartame did not affect working memory, consuming a high-aspartame diet resulted in participants exhibiting irritable moods, more depression, and poorer performance on spatial orientation tests.[321] One component of aspartame, the amino acid phenylalanine, is sold as a supplement and naturally occurs in many foods such as milk and meat. It is harmful to people who suffer from phenylketonuria (PKU), a rare condition where they cannot metabolize it well.

Other substances such as cysteine, an amino acid used to extend shelf life, and casein, a protein compound, are also added to foods. The former has been shown to cause neurological disease, and the latter, neuroinflammation and delayed processing speed.[322, 323] Casein is found in milk products, especially cheeses, and is often seen on labels in the form of sodium caseinate. Sodium caseinate is found in margarine, whipped toppings, and bakery glazes and also in seemingly healthy foods such as protein bars and infant formula.

- *Excitotoxins*

Many different types of substances are added to foods, and some of them can have detrimental effects. One such group is excitotoxins, which stimulate neuron receptors and facilitate brain communication. When consumed in large quantities, however, these excitotoxins overtax the neurons, weakening them and resulting in cell death. Monosodium glutamate (MSG) is one such excitotoxin and is the powdered form of glutamate or glutamic acid. While glutamate is necessary for normal brain function, an excessive amount can lead to cognitive issues. A 2018 review of the effects of MSG concluded that possible toxic effects of MSG may have been underestimated and include nervous system disorders, obesity, disruptions in fat metabolism, liver damage, and reproductive malfunctions.[324] MSG is currently allowed as a flavor enhancer by the FDA and must be listed on ingredient labels. It is found in many processed foods such as soups, potato chips, meat, frozen foods, and salad dressings.

While small amounts of excitotoxins are acceptable by the FDA, the impact they have on any given person depends on genetics, amounts consumed, prescription medications being taken, and other health conditions. Any single toxin may not cause significant damage, but collectively, many small harms can add up to substantial negative impacts. It is important to avoid letting various toxins build up in the body, thereby increasing the toxic body burden.

- *Food Coloring and Additives*

Food colorings have been studied to see if they pose a toxic or otherwise adverse effect on the human body. Chemically derived colors, flavors, and additives have been linked to adverse health effects in children and adults, impacting the nervous and endocrine systems, which directly affect brain health. There are many types of food colorings, and some are naturally derived, such as riboflavin, a B vitamin that has an orange-yellow color or red coloring from beets. Other food colorings are chemically derived and have been shown to cause a range of reactions, including hyperactivity, changes in the nervous system, and allergic reactions that increase inflammation in the body.[325, 326, 327] Synthetic food colorings have also been linked to endocrine issues.[328] A 2019 study on the biological effects of food coloring states that "the overall results would support the idea that a high chronic intake of these additives throughout the entire life is not advisable."[329]

- *Food Packaging*

Another way we may be exposed to toxins is through our food packaging. Whether it is cans that have bisphenol A in their lining or plastics that release harmful chemicals in our food and beverages (discussed later in the Plastics section), repeated exposure may disrupt our hormonal system and add to our toxic body burden.[330] These adverse exposures may not only affect the individual but also can be passed down through genes to the next generation.[331]

Phthalates are chemicals used in manufacturing to make plastics more pliable. Used mainly in food packaging and consumer products (children's toys, medical devices, furniture, PVC plumbing, vinyl flooring, wall coverings, detergents and household cleaners, etc.), phthalates can be found almost everywhere, including indoor dust and air, cosmetics, food, and our bodies. On labels, they may be listed as "fragrance" or "flavor." These substances are known by various names[332] and have been shown to be harmful to humans, even in utero. Some studies show that mothers who have been exposed to phthalates have children with lower cognition scores and delays in motor development and language.[333, 334] They are also endocrine disruptors and have an adverse effect on multiple organ systems, especially in children.[335, 336]

A study done on elderly subjects found a correlation between exposure to phthalates and lower scores on immediate and delayed recall tests.[337] More research is needed on the effects of phthalates on adults and older populations. While phthalates have been regulated to a wide degree in the United States and Europe, they are pervasive and take a long time to break down, so longer-term effects are unknown.

- *Pesticides and Herbicides*

Chemicals sprayed on foods for both growing and harvesting have become problematic, as they contribute daily to the total toxic body burden as well as potentially impacting cognitive function. Different types of chemicals are used in growing and harvesting cycles to ward off insects, to improve the look of fruits and vegetables, and for drying out crops before harvesting.

Studies dating back to 1998 show that Mexican children exposed to a mixture of agricultural chemicals showed adverse effects on motor skills, memory, attention, and learning.[338] A meta-analysis of seven studies in 2016 "suggested a positive association between pesticide exposure and AD, confirming the hypothesis that pesticide exposure is a risk factor for AD."[339]

Revealing events in recent years have exposed the damage caused by the commercial weed-killer Roundup, whose active ingredient is glyphosate. This product is commonly sprayed on crops such as wheat and hops to dry them out, thereby expediting the harvesting process. In the past several years, lawsuits against Roundup's manufacturer, Monsanto, have accused the chemical company of ignoring health problems caused by glyphosate, including non-Hodgkin lymphoma and other forms of cancer.[340] We have reason to believe that glyphosate also adversely affects the brain and may lead to dementia.[341]

The gut and the brain are connected via the vagus nerve, and nerve signals are sent back and forth constantly. The gut produces about 75 percent of the brain's neurotransmitters. Glyphosate harms the gut microbiome because it kills beneficial bacteria and adversely affects the body's immune system. The immune system, specifically the innate immune system, plays a critical role in Alzheimer's disease. When the body is exposed to toxins, it causes inflammation and sets the stage for "toxin-related Alzheimer's." Recent research shows that glyphosate crosses the blood-brain barrier and increases pro-inflammatory cytokines in blood plasma.[342]

Glyphosate also has the ability to bind with and hold onto minerals, potentially creating demineralization in the body.[343] Minerals are critical for hundreds of processes in the body; sodium, potassium, magnesium, calcium, and copper are responsible for the transmission of nerve impulses, which may impact brain functioning.

- *Trans Fats*

Trans fats, often listed as hydrogenated or partially hydrogenated oil on food labels, have been shown to cause dementia. People with higher levels of trans fats in their blood were 50 to 75 percent more likely to develop Alzheimer's disease or dementia.[344] Among the foods most likely to contribute to trans fats intake in the study were pastries, margarine, candies and caramels, nondairy creamers, ice cream, and rice crackers. Despite these findings, the FDA still allowed foods with less than 0.5 grams of trans fats to be labeled as containing zero grams of trans fats. By January 2020, U.S. food manufacturers were finally no longer allowed to sell foods containing partially hydrogenated oil.

Home and Work Environments

Indoor environments can be unhealthier than the outside for a variety of reasons. Our homes and workplaces tend to be closed spaces where air may not circulate freely. Dirt and other residues can be tracked in on shoes, and home cleaning and personal products often contain harmful chemicals and fragrances. New furniture and other manufactured products may emit odors for weeks, releasing potentially hazardous chemicals into the air (e.g., new sofa, rug, or car smell).

While it's essential to pay attention to the sources of environmental exposure, it is also critical to know when we are exposed. Fetuses, young children, and teens develop at such a rapid rate that chemicals can have added harmful health effects. In one study, children from households where their mothers used toxic chemicals in products such as household cleaners showed delayed learning and lower scores on a test of cognitive development.[345] Plasticizers (additives that soften plastic, making it resilient and elastic, including bisphenol A and phthalates) can cross the fetoplacental barrier and be observed to result in growth retardation and neurological damage.[346]

Most chemicals used in home products are not tested for safety, and in the United States, they are not regulated for safety or toxicity.

When the word "fragrance" or "perfume" is listed on a label, the product is considered proprietary, so the consumer cannot know the actual ingredients. Added fragrances can contain hundreds of harmful chemicals that get into the body and affect the normal workings of the endocrine and immune systems. They can also cause difficulty with breathing and trigger asthma attacks. Synthetic chemicals that we breathe in are especially harmful to children and pregnant women.

Volatile organic compounds (VOCs) are gases emitted from certain solids and liquids and contribute to indoor pollution. VOCs are contained in many products, including paints, varnishes, and waxes; cleaning and disinfecting solutions and dry-cleaned clothing; cosmetics; degreasers; and hobby products. These products can release organic compounds while in use and, to some degree, when they are stored. According to the EPA, VOCs can cause headaches, loss of coordination, dizziness, memory impairment, fatigue, and damage to the liver, kidney, and central nervous system.[347] Formaldehyde is one of the most common VOCs, and there is evidence that inhaled formaldehyde negatively affects learning and memory capacity.[348]

Whether measuring outdoor or indoor pollutants such as nitrogen dioxide (primarily from the combustion of fossil fuels like coal, gas, and oil) and black carbon, both were predictive of decreased cognitive function in children.[349, 350] A 2018 study in India reported that those individuals exposed to indoor air pollution from the use of biomass fuels and coals for household purposes were found to have a twofold likelihood of having cognitive impairment.[351]

One other source of potential toxins in the home is nonstick pans that are coated with Teflon, which is made from PFAS (per- and polyfluoroalkyl substances). PFAS are chemicals that are also used to make products stain-resistant and waterproof, and the chemical is released when foods in the pans are cooked at high temperatures. As the coating becomes scratched and worn, more of the chemicals are released. Some microwave popcorn bags, fast-food wrappers, rain jackets, and other consumer products use these chemicals' "nonstick" properties. PFAS and their byproducts accumulate in the environment and may harm human health (see the Water section for more information).

Personal Care Products
Personal care products and their ingredients are not regulated in the United States. Under the 1976 Toxic Substances Control Act, products that are rubbed, lathered, and sprayed onto our bodies require no testing for safety or toxicity before going to market. We do not know the extent of their reproductive risks, potential developmental issues in children, cancer risks, or risk of endocrine disorders.[352, 353] The ingredients that we know do have those effects have not been removed or banned.

Since 1976, only 11 chemicals have been removed from cosmetics in the United States. The European Union has restricted 2,400 chemicals in their products since the 1970s, most of which are still used in the United States. Many personal products contain endocrine-disrupting chemicals (EDCs) that can alter hormone levels in the body. Others may contain preservatives, coloring, and metals such as lead and mercury. Teens are a prime audience for cosmetic and personal care products; they use more of them than any other demographic, exposing them to potentially harmful chemicals over many decades. While these products on their own have not been shown to cause dementia, long-term exposure to harmful ingredients contributes to the cumulative toxic burden on our bodies.

Plastics
The use of plastic in products and the environment has increased exponentially over the past several decades. They are found nearly everywhere, from our food sources to the oceans, in the air and household dust, and in human organs, glands, and placenta. Humans are typically exposed through ingestion or inhalation. Not only are plas-

tics ubiquitous, but their compositional parts are potentially so small (called microplastics or nanoplastics) that they now have the ability to cross the blood-brain barrier. In doing so, they pose a new and unique threat to the body and the brain.

We are just learning about the harmful effects of microplastics, which are 5 millimeters or less in length (smaller than a sesame seed). These can break down even further to nanoplastics, which are small enough to enter the body's cells and tissues. A liter of bottled water, for example, can contain 240,000 of these tiny particles. Early research has shown some adverse health effects from chemicals in plastics, including infertility, cancer, metabolic disorders, and ADD/ADHD.[354, 355, 356, 357] Few studies have been done on humans, and more research is needed.

Research on rats, however, has shown that adding microplastics to their drinking water caused behavioral changes as well as alterations in immune markers in liver and brain tissues. Particularly noteworthy was that the changes differed depending on age, indicating a possible age-dependent effect.[358] Another study exposed mice to orally consumed polystyrene or a mixture of polymer microspheres. Not only were microplastics found in the brain, liver, and kidneys, but metabolic differences were observed in the colon, brain, and liver.[359] A study on honeybees that exposed them to different types of microplastics for two days showed impaired learning and memory and raised concerns about potential mechanical, cellular, and biochemical damage that microplastics may cause to the central nervous system.[360]

Studies have shown that microplastics alter human "microbial colonic community composition."[361] An encouraging finding is that bifidobacterium *infantis*, a probiotic that regulates the intestinal microbiota, has been shown to break down polypropylene, which is generally used as synthetic plastic.[362] Another study on mice exposed to nanopolystyrene shows that the nanoplastic caused microbial alteration and metabolic disorders and possible immune dysregulation.

Bifidobacterium breve M-16V, found in the intestines of infants, may possibly alleviate the gut microbiota dysbiosis.[363] Fermented foods are good sources of bifidobacteria, including milk kefir, sourdough bread, sauerkraut, kimchi, and other fermented vegetables.

Water

United States public drinking water supplies are considered some of the safest in the world and are regulated by the EPA to protect against both naturally occurring and man-made contaminants. According to the EPA, drinking water reasonably may be expected to contain at least small amounts of contaminants, some of which are harmless and others that may be harmful if consumed at certain levels.[364]

The main categories of contaminants are microorganisms (e.g., E. coli, giardia, and noroviruses), inorganic chemicals (e.g., lead, arsenic, copper, fluoride, nitrates, and nitrites), organic chemicals (e.g., atrazine, glyphosate, trichloroethylene, and tetrachloroethylene), and disinfection by-products (e.g., chloroform). Another category of contaminants called PFAS (per- and polyfluoroalkyl substances) or "forever chemicals" are widely used, and their components break down very slowly over time. They have been found in humans and animals, various food products, water, fish, and soil. In April 2024, the EPA announced a new rule limiting PFAS in public drinking water systems, giving utilities five years to comply.

The National Institutes of Health (NIH) outlined the risk of PFAS in terms of the number of chemicals, repeated and widespread exposure, and bioaccumulation.[365] Effects of PFAS on the human body include hormone, immune, lipid, and insulin disruption; liver disease and cancer; and reproductive and developmental problems.[366] More research is needed on the impact of PFAS on the nervous system, but it is clear from the above associations that cognition may be compromised.

It is important for everyone to be aware of the quality of their own drinking water. The Consumer Confidence Report, an annual drinking water quality report, is required by the EPA and available online. Households using private well water are responsible for testing and maintaining the safety of their drinking water, which may be contaminated with microorganisms, heavy metals, nitrate and nitrite, organic chemicals including pesticides, and radionuclides such as radon and uranium. These homeowners should test their well water regularly using an accredited laboratory.

For concerns about water quality in the home — or even simply to improve the taste of tap water — one approach is to filter drinking water using one or more of the available technologies. Depending on what specific contaminants are of most concern, available space, anticipated usage, and cost, options include a whole-house filter, under-the-sink or faucet filters, or water pitchers. For more serious contamination concerns, reverse osmosis filters remove the highest amount of contaminants (including vital minerals), and they often reduce water flow rates and may change the pH of the water. Other options may be available, such as carbon filters. Regardless of which approach is used, all filters should have a stamp or seal identifying which specific contaminants it removes, such as lead, chlorine, or PFAS, and be NSF/ANSI-certified.

Preventing Exposure to Toxins

The ability to reduce exposure to toxic chemicals is dependent on the types of toxins to which we are exposed, where we are exposed, and the frequency of exposure. Here are some suggestions to avoid common toxins.

Air
- Use an air purifier with a HEPA filter if you are known to have allergies or react to dust.[367] Some air purifiers can now kill microorganisms, including mold.

- Allow new furniture/carpeting to off-gas outside the home whenever possible, or keep windows open with new furniture and carpeting.[368]
- Remove the plastic cover from dry cleaning and allow clothes to air out before putting them in the closet.
- Don't burn candles, wood stoves, fireplaces, or gas appliances in your home.
- Properly ventilate your home by opening windows and turning on fans when you cook or shower.
- Use a dehumidifier to keep humidity levels between 30 and 50 percent. Higher humidity levels can exacerbate upper respiratory conditions.
- Don't inhale around idling vehicles.

Electromagnetic Frequencies
- Several companies sell products that claim to protect against the effects of cell phone radiation. We recommend reading their research to see which may be appropriate for you.
- Charge your phone at night in a room other than your bedroom.
- Do not stand in front of a microwave oven when it is on, and use it sparingly.
- Keep your cell phone away from your head and your brain, and never have it stowed next to the skin. Use the phone on speaker mode.

Food
- Go to the Environmental Working Group website (ewg.org) for a list of the "Clean Fifteen" and "Dirty Dozen" to know which fruits and vegetables are most likely to have pesticide and herbicide residue; these should be bought organic whenever possible. Rinse all fruits and vegetables with water before consuming, whether they are organic or not, and, for added safety, use a fruit and vegetable

wash to remove bacteria and other toxins.
- Read labels to look for artificial flavors (including "natural flavors"), colors, sweeteners, and preservatives.
- For those foods consumed in greater amounts and fed to young children such as milk or eggs, buy organic if your budget allows.
- Meats and poultry that are grass-fed and/or organic result in food containing more nutrients and fewer hormones and toxins. Look for labeling that states no antibiotics or hormones were used.
- Consume fewer foods from boxes, bags, and those that come in plastic packaging.
- Try to store food in glass containers or wrap foods in parchment paper or soy wax paper before storing or freezing in plastic bags.
- If using plastic storage products, look for those that are BPA-free and microwave safe.

Home and Work Environments
- Use natural cleaning products like white vinegar, water, and sea salt to scrub sticky surfaces, and add lemon juice or essential lavender oil for fragrance.[369] Other natural products made with essential oils may also be highly effective as they contain antibacterial, antiviral, and antifungal properties.[370]
- If the temperature outside is comfortable and you do not suffer from severe pollen allergies, open your windows for at least 15 minutes every day.
- Remove the artificial air fresheners in your home — aerosols, plug-ins, diffusers, carpet powders — and any products that have synthetic ingredients. Look for 100 percent organic cleaning products and nontoxic candles, incense, and laundry detergent.
- Dust and vacuum weekly with a HEPA filter vacuum because household dust has been found to contain hundreds of chemicals that come from products we use in our homes every day. Children and household pets have been shown to have the highest levels of many chemicals in their bodies because they are on the floor where

dust collects and adheres to toys, fingers, and paws.
- Try to buy clothing with natural fibers and that do not require dry cleaning.
- Take off your shoes before entering a home to avoid tracking in pesticides and other potential toxins.
- Discard worn/scratched nonstick cookware and look for brands that are PFA-free. Consider using stainless steel, ceramic, or cast iron. Discontinue using nonstick cookware purchased before 2015.
- When you smell car or truck exhaust or air that is otherwise contaminated, try to hold your breath or cover your mouth and nose until the exposure has passed. When refueling at gas stations, try not to inhale vapors.

Personal Care Products
- Be aware of what you put on your skin. Try to use fewer products overall, especially during pregnancy. Consult apps below to avoid products containing toxic chemicals. Read labels to avoid products that contain fragrance or perfume, even in body sprays and aftershaves for boys and men. Avoid oxybenzone, retinyl palmitate, or retinol in sunscreens and lip products. Avoid products with parabens, ethylene glycol, aluminum, and phthalates.
- Choose water-based nail polish without acetone, toluene, and formaldehyde; several brands are now for sale.
- Tampons and feminine care products that are 100 percent organic cotton and are free of chlorine, phthalates, and pesticides are available. Check your products on the Environment Working Group website or in the apps below.
- Apps that list ingredients in personal care products also rate their safety risks. Use apps such as Yuka, Think Dirty, and the EWG's Healthy Living to choose safer options.

Plastics
- Avoid plastic packaging when possible, especially plastic water

bottles.
- Don't microwave or heat food in plastic containers.
- Use glass or stainless steel containers for food storage.
- Do not drink out of plastic bottles that have been exposed to heat, and avoid them if possible.
- Choose stainless steel, silicone, and wood kitchen tools.

Water
- Drink filtered water, and use a glass, stainless steel, or silicone bottle.
- If you have well water, make sure to have it tested.
- If you have municipal water, read the annual test results provided by your local water company, and choose a filter that addresses the highest contaminants.

Treatments for Toxins

As toxins have become more prevalent in our environment, increasing our toxic body burden, some environmental scientists and physicians suggest that a daily detoxification regimen might be advisable in addition to taking the preventive steps outlined above.

As previously mentioned, each person is unique, and some individuals are more sensitive or susceptible to toxins due to age, health, lifestyle, levels and consistency of exposure, or epigenetics where certain genes may be turned on or off due to stress, trauma, infection, or other conditions. Before beginning any detoxification protocol, diagnostic testing should be conducted to determine the type and level of toxins and/or mycotoxins that may be present.

The liver and kidneys are primarily responsible for ridding the body of toxins, so supporting these organs is paramount. There are various ways to do this, including increasing hydration, adding specific foods to the diet, and using herbs such as nettle, dandelion, milk thistle, and chlorella as teas or in capsule form. Working with a health coach or integrative doctor is recommended because specific herbs support the various organs and detoxification processes. Sweating regularly during exercise or in a sauna is also an effective way to release toxins naturally. Detoxification programs typically start with a healthy diet, optimizing the gut microbiome and elimination system, adequate hydration, and a regular exercise program to make sure pathways in the body are functioning well. Home water and air filtration systems may also be helpful. If the body's toxic levels have become too high, however, further intervention may be needed.

There are a few laboratories in the United States that provide broad spectrum testing for environmental toxins and mycotoxins, which should be ordered by a doctor who can interpret the results and suggest treatment protocols. Because this is a relatively new area of testing, diagnosis, treatment, and finding the right doctor may be challenging. Functional medicine, integrative doctors, naturopaths, and other holistic practitioners may have experience with detoxification and/or specialize in specific conditions such as Lyme disease or mold toxicity. See Finding Qualified Healthcare Professionals for more information about finding a qualified medical or dental practitioner.

Depending on the particular type of toxin or group of toxins (e.g., mold toxicity, heavy metals, etc.), therapy options may be diverse and multifaceted and require a practitioner with expertise to design an effective treatment program. Toxic effects initially may be limited to a specific area of the body or become systemic, creating inflammation throughout the body. Additional approaches for treating these effects may include the use of red light therapy, infrared saunas, ionic foot baths, hydrogen therapy, BioMats, glutathione therapy, or binders such as zeolite, bentonite clay, or activated charcoal. It may be necessary to try one approach or multiple approaches at once and fine-tune as needed, so finding and working with an experienced practitioner is paramount.

Conclusion

Due to the proliferation of chemicals and industrial by-products in our air and our environment, our toxic exposures have increased exponentially over the past several decades. Depending on where we live, our access to clean air and water, our diet and personal care products, and our genes, we may have multiple exposures that accumulate over time and eventually overwhelm our systems, resulting in a "toxic body burden." In the future, we may want to adopt a daily detoxification regimen to offset the levels of toxins in our systems. In the meantime, we can all take steps to reduce our toxic exposure and improve lifestyle habits around nutrition, sleep, stress, and exercise to give our bodies every opportunity to stay healthy.

9

Heavy Metal Toxicity

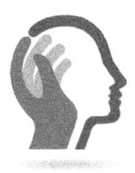

HEAVY METALS ARE FOUND IN THE NATURAL WORLD, and some, like copper, iron, manganese, and zinc, are important for the human body to function optimally. Small quantities of these heavy metals are required to keep us healthy. When we have too much or the wrong type of metals accumulating in our body, we may experience health issues. Some heavy metals are known to be neurotoxins (poisonous to our nerves and brain), and others can damage the kidneys, contribute to cardiovascular disease, and cause cancer. The symptoms of mercury toxicity, for example, mimic those of Alzheimer's disease. It is for this reason that we focus on heavy metals separately. This chapter describes how we are exposed to heavy metals, why they can be dangerous, and how we can remove them from our bodies to prevent memory loss or lessen the toxic load that the body has accumulated.

The human body is a miraculous set of systems that processes the food we eat and distributes nutrients to every cell where it is combined with oxygen to efficiently and effectively produce all the energy needed for our daily functions and necessary repair. One of these many systems identifies and eliminates the by-products and waste our cells produce as well as monitors foreign threats and invaders.

Detoxification is a process built into the human body where chemicals and other substances are processed primarily in the liver and eliminated from the body through our sweat, urine, and stool. When we ingest, breathe, or absorb through the skin substances that are not healthy, over time, our immune and detoxification systems can become overburdened and cease to work properly. Toxins can damage tissue and cause hormone disruption, altering chemical signaling in the body.[371] Our overall health and mental well-being depends on how well all of our systems function together. It is important to understand the specific factors that impair this function, and one of these is the accumulation of heavy metals.

Consider a labor strike or a bad winter storm where garbage is not picked up for days; it accumulates, produces a foul smell, and clutters the entrances to homes and apartments, making them a less comfortable place to live. This also happens in the body, often without our knowledge and awareness.

What Are Heavy Metals?

Heavy metals are a group of substances that have a relatively high density, are toxic at low levels (parts per billion — ppb), and tend to accumulate in the environment and in our bodies. Heavy metals to be aware of are antimony, arsenic, bismuth, cadmium, cerium, chromium, cobalt, copper, gallium, gold, iron, lead, manganese, mercury, nickel, platinum, silver, tellurium, thallium, tin, uranium, vanadium, and zinc. Some like manganese, copper, zinc, and iron are essential for certain biological processes, but only in small amounts. In larger amounts, they, too, can become toxic. Other heavy metals like lead, arsenic, mercury, cadmium, nickel, and aluminum are harmful and neurotoxic, especially if they build up in the body over time.

Dangers of Heavy Metal Toxicity

Heavy metal (HM) toxicity can lower energy levels, impact the composition of our blood, and damage the functioning of the brain, lungs, kidney, liver, and other important organs.[372] HM toxicity can also mimic certain diseases and can accumulate individually or in combination to increase the risk for a range of neurological diseases such as Alzheimer's, multiple sclerosis, Parkinson's, Guillain-Barré syndrome, Huntington's disease, autism, and ALS (Lou Gehrig's disease or MND — motor neuron disease).

Those with HM toxicity may also exhibit personality and behavioral changes such as depression, hostility, and mood swings.[373] Over time, the risk of developing any of these conditions, including Alzheimer's and dementia, increases with the buildup of toxins in the body. It is the total accumulation, more than chronological age, that increases the chances of developing dementia due to toxic exposures.

How Heavy Metals Accumulate in the Body

When heavy metals cannot be eliminated by the body's natural detoxification processes, they are absorbed. The body usually stores them first in relatively stable places like bones and fat. (Mercury has a particular affinity for fatty tissues.) When the body runs out of the most stable places to store toxins, it sends them to the organs, including the brain, the liver, and the kidneys.

When all fixed locations are full and heavy metals and other toxins are still entering the body at a rate faster than the body can excrete them, we say the body has exceeded its "toxic body burden."[374] As toxicity levels increase, normal function is compromised, and symptoms (see the list later in this section) become more obvious. HM toxicity is a result of exposure and lack of ability to clear toxins from the body. This can be the result of poor diet, nonrestorative sleep, dehydration, lack of exercise, poor stress management, and even genetic factors.

People with the ApoE4 gene, which is known to increase the risk for developing Alzheimer's disease, have a reduced ability to excrete heavy metals, thus increasing the risk of developing Alzheimer's symptoms at an earlier age. However, being diligent about diet, sleep, hydration, exercise, and stress management can help to offset the genetic risk.

Heavy Metals That Are Problematic for the Body and Brain

Lead

Lead has been shown to be neurotoxic, especially for children exposed to lead-based paint. Another source is lead found in pipes. As the danger of lead toxicity has become more evident, the Centers for Disease Control and Prevention (CDC) has steadily lowered the threshold for blood lead levels (BLLs) considered dangerous in children by 90 percent, from 60 µg/dL to 3.5 µg/dL.[375] We no longer have leaded gasoline for this reason. More recently, the impact of lead in the water of Flint, Michigan (2014–2015), from old lead pipes resulted in residents experiencing a range of health issues, including a precipitous drop in third-grade proficiency test scores.[376]

Several studies have found an association between higher levels of lead in the body and declines in cognitive performance.[377, 378, 379] A concern also exists that even a low-level accumulation of lead over a lifetime, as experienced by older adults, may be harmful to cognitive performance. Researchers Walter F. Stewart and Brian S. Schwartz posit that what is thought to be "normal" cognitive decline due to age may in fact be due to an accumulation of neurotoxins, such as lead.[380]

More recently, lead and cadmium have been found in dark chocolate at sometimes harmful levels. See the chapter on Nutrition and Supplements for more information.

Mercury

Mercury is a nonessential metal that affects the function and development of the central nervous system. Fifty to one hundred times more neurotoxic than lead, mercury accumulates in the brain, the thyroid, the adrenals, the liver, and the heart. It also alters the body's immune functions, exacerbating autoimmune reactivity. Mercury collects in the fatty layer of the cell membrane. It changes how the cell appears to the immune system, and the immune system attacks it as if it were a foreign invader.

Mercury can be a problem even in utero. It has been shown to have widespread distribution in the fetuses of mothers who have amalgam (silver) fillings in place and in breast milk. This amounts to approximately 630,000 babies born every year at risk of developmental problems because of prenatal mercury exposure.[381] For those who are exposed to lead pipes and lead paint as children, mercury may be an even bigger problem.

Since all heavy metals use the same detoxification pathway, the presence of lead and other heavy metals obstructs and delays the excretion of mercury (and all heavy metals). According to neurosurgeon Russell Blaylock, MD, mercury inflicts serious damage and is related to a wide range of neurological pathologies. For example, mercury:

- Poisons enzymes that are important for energy production[382]
- Interrupts the process by which growing nerves develop protective covering (myelin sheath)[383]
- Activates immune-excitotoxicity,[384] which:
  » Dramatically increases the generation of free radicals
  » Accelerates atherosclerosis (hardening of the arteries)
  » Generally depresses the immune system
  » Damages and kills nerve cells by increasing inflammation
  » Lowers levels of glutathione (useful in detoxifying)
  » Raises glutamate (an excitatory neurotransmitter) to toxic levels
  » Severely damages the endothelia (lining), especially of blood vessels

When the lining of blood vessels is damaged, it may lead to further disease in the body, including diabetes mellitus, hypertension, rheumatoid arthritis, lupus, and coronary artery disease (which can lead to vascular dementia). All this activity in the vascular system limits blood flow to the organs and tissues of the body (including the brain), which diminishes both the nourishment and the natural daily detoxifying functions the bloodstream makes possible.

Sources of Mercury
If you grew up or live in an industrialized country or area, you almost certainly have been exposed to mercury from a variety of sources. If you are over the age of 30, you have likely encountered mercury through impure air or water, eating large fish such as tuna or swordfish, or in your dental treatment. For many years, "silver" amalgam fillings were the most widely used dental restorations, and their composition is 50 percent mercury.

"Silver" Fillings
In addition to containing mercury, silver amalgam fillings also contain silver, zinc, and sometimes even lead. Silver fillings present in the mouth for years can break down through chewing, grinding of teeth, tooth polishing, and decay. However, by the time a filling has been in a tooth for 25 years, the amount of mercury drops by up to 80 percent. That is because, in addition to fragmenting into nanoparticles that might be ingested, mercury fillings regularly emit mercury vapor. Even the American Dental Association acknowledges that mercury off-gasses continuously, and we breathe that vapor into our lungs up to 1,750 times per day.[385] The exposure is particularly high and dangerous for those with several fillings, especially if they were placed after 1970 when amalgams were high in copper. In addition, people who have both gold and mercury amalgam in their mouths experience a high galvanic reaction between the various metals, which exacerbates the effect of the mercury, especially when the mouth is an acidic environment.

Power Plants
Mercury in the environment can find its ways into lakes or waterways. Bacteria convert it into methylmercury, a more potent toxin. Coal-fired power plants spew tons of mercury into the air every year and

are responsible for approximately 50 percent of human-caused mercury emissions. According to the Environmental Protection Agency website, the 1,400 coal- and oil-fired electric generating units at 600 power plants in the United States "emit harmful pollutants, including mercury, non-mercury metallic toxics, acid gases, and organic air toxics such as dioxin."[386]

Large Fish
Mercury (in the form of methylmercury) is found in fish and shellfish, which are readily available for human consumption. Mercury increases in concentration with each step up the food chain. Large predator fish eat many smaller fish and can have mercury levels over one million times that of the surrounding water, and people who consume fish with high mercury levels are at risk of serious health problems.[387]

In 2004, the FDA advised that young children, pregnant women, and nursing women avoid four fish (shark, swordfish, king mackerel, and tilefish) that contain high levels of mercury.[388] Another fish with dangerously high levels of mercury is tuna, a fish often used for sushi, tuna fish salad, or grilled as a steak. It is wise to confine consumption to smaller fish that are not in the ocean for as long a time. See Environmental Working Group's Good Seafood Guide (https://www.ewg.org/research/ewgs-good-seafood-guide) for more information on fish that are safe to consume.

Vaccines
Flu vaccines that have multiple doses in the vial may contain small amounts of mercury as a preservative, and even so-called thimerosal-free vaccines can have trace amounts.

Other Sources of Mercury Exposure
In addition to these broad categories, certain types of industrial jobs bring people into contact with heavy metals, and industrial accidents have exposed workers to high levels of heavy metal vapors and other

by-products. Personal care products that lighten the skin and other cosmetics and pharmaceuticals have been found to contain mercury. Mercury used to be included in paints, wallpaper, paste, antiseptics (Mercurochrome), and even in birth control products. It has now been removed from these products, but you may have had exposure sometime in the past.

Signs and Symptoms of Mercury Toxicity
Exposure to mercury can cause a wide range of symptoms and, in some cases, mimic those of Alzheimer's disease or increase the risk for AD.[389]

Questions to determine the potential risk of mercury toxicity:
- Do you now — or did you ever — have silver/mercury amalgam fillings?
- Do you have any other metal fillings or crowns in your mouth?
- Are you allergic to any jewelry (e.g., nickel)?
- Do you ever have a metallic taste in your mouth?
- Do you eat a lot of seafood — especially tuna, swordfish, and other large fish?
- Do you suffer from any chronic disease?
- Have you ever had a dental filling removed or replaced without the protection of a rubber dam, high-speed suction, or oxygen over your nose?
- Do you experience any of the following symptoms?

Most common signs and symptoms of heavy metal poisoning:
- Alcohol intolerance
- Allergies
- Anxiety and irritability
- Brain fog
- Chronic unexplained pain
- Coated tongue
- Cold hands and feet
- Dark circles under the eyes
- Depression
- Digestive problems

- Extreme fatigue
- Frequent colds and flu
- Headaches
- Inability to lose weight
- Insomnia
- Intolerance to medications
- Loss of memory and forgetfulness
- Low body temperature
- Metallic taste in mouth
- Muscle and joint pain
- Muscle tics or twitches
- Muscle tremors
- Night sweats
- Parasites
- Proneness to mood swings
- Proneness to rashes
- Sensitive teeth
- Sensitivity to smells like tobacco smoke, perfumes, paint fumes, and chemical odors
- Skin problems
- Small black spots on the gums
- Sore or receding gums
- Tingling in the extremities
- Unsteady gait
- Vitamin and mineral deficiency

Aluminum

Aluminum is the third most common element found on the earth's crust. It finds its way into the body by inhalation, ingestion, and dermal contact. Sources of exposure are drinking water, food, beverages, aluminum-heavy drugs, personal care products, and cooking pans. Aluminum is naturally present in many foods such as baked goods, processed foods, some herbs, and hot drinks (cocoa, coffee, tea).

Too much aluminum in the body affects virtually every organ as well as bones and the nervous system.[390] Symptoms of aluminum toxicity may include nausea, mouth ulcers, skin ulcers, skin rashes, vomiting, diarrhea, and arthritic pain.[391] The World Health Organization stated in 1997 that aluminum exposure was a risk factor for the onset of Alzheimer disease in humans. In 2010, the WHO reduced a tolerable weekly intake of aluminum per person from 7 mg/kg of body weight down to just 1 mg/kg, but with the pushback from industry, compromised on 2 mg/kg of body weight.[392] Adverse effects on the nervous system include loss of memory, problems with balance, and loss of coordination.

People suffering from kidney diseases find it difficult to eliminate aluminum from the body, resulting in aluminum accumulation that can lead to bone and brain damage. Categorizing aluminum as a neurotoxin has been controversial for many years, with much of the research being performed and funded by the industry itself. However, there is evidence that aluminum can build up in the body, affect cellular processes, and impact those areas of the brain that are responsible for memory.[393] Aluminum can cross the blood-brain barrier and accumulate in the brain in small amounts over time. Studies of people whose drinking water contained a high level of aluminum (more than 100 mcg/L) had an average of three times greater risk for developing Alzheimer's disease.[394] In addition to aluminum being found in the brains of people with AD,[395, 396] it also accumulates more quickly in the brains of older versus middle-aged adults[397] and seems to be concentrated most in the hippocampus, the area responsible for short-term memory.

Arsenic

Arsenic contaminations have occurred through both natural and man-made sources. The smelting process can release arsenic into the air and soil and can affect the quality of surface water through groundwater ejection and runoff. Paints, dyes, soaps, metals, semiconductors, and drugs may contain arsenic. Pesticides, fertilizers, and animal feeding operations also can release arsenic to the environment.

The inorganic forms of arsenic are more dangerous to human health. They are highly carcinogenic and can cause cancer of lungs, liver, bladder, and skin. Humans are exposed to arsenic by means of air, food, and water. Drinking water contaminated with arsenic is one of the major causes for arsenic toxicity in more than 30 countries in the world. According to the American Cancer Society, foods highest in arsenic are seafood, rice, rice cereal (and other rice products), mushrooms, and poultry, although many other foods, including some fruit juices, can also contain arsenic.[398]

Other Heavy Metals

Other metals that impact the brain include beryllium, cadmium, nickel, and chromium. These metals are absorbed into the body through food, air pollution, medications, vaccines, pesticides, spermicide, and some beauty and personal care products. Because heavy metals build up in the body in bone, organs, and fatty tissues, they may cause different symptoms. As previously mentioned, they produce oxidative stress and chronic inflammation leading to irritability, disturbed sleep, memory issues, immune dysfunction, gastrointestinal issues, headaches, tremors, and coordination problems.[399]

Heavy Metals Testing

Someone who is experiencing one or more of the symptoms listed above may want to be tested for heavy metal toxicity to determine the extent of the body's exposure. Most integrative and functional medicine doctors routinely test for heavy metals in their practices. Different doctors may prefer blood, urine, hair, or stool tests. Although mercury is the most commonly tested heavy metal, similar tests are used for the others.

The single most common mercury test for many years has been a urine challenge test. Some doctors recommend a two-step testing process: The first step involves testing heavy metal levels in urine over a 6-, 12-, or 24-hour period. The second step covers the same amount of collection time but introduces a chelation drug that binds with the heavy metals in the bloodstream, creating a compound the body removes when urinating. The medication — dimercapto propanesulfonate (DMPS) — is given either orally dimercaptopropane sulfonic acid (DMSA) or through an IV along with the antioxidant glutathione.

The first specimen, collected without the addition of any chelating medium, indicates how much mercury the body is eliminating on its own. (A mercury level of under 4 mcg is considered a healthy level of excretion.) The second specimen shows how much more the body can excrete when it has some kind of assistance.

If the amount of mercury in the second specimen is several times greater than in the first specimen, say 8 to 12 mcg, it may indicate that the tissues in the body are carrying a substantial amount of these metals and that they are unable to excrete them without significant additional help in the form of a detoxification regimen.

High mercury or other heavy metal levels in the urine should alert the practitioner to the need for a pre-detox protocol to ensure that the body's evacuation channels — skin, liver, colon, and kidneys — are functioning efficiently. Strengthening the channels of elimination should be a first step in treatment so that during detoxification, these heavy metals are not reabsorbed elsewhere in the body, such as the brain and nervous system.

Ridding the Body of Heavy Metals

One important step to ridding the body of heavy metals is to stop adding to the body's toxic burden by avoiding exposure in the first place. This includes being aware of what may be brought into the house (e.g., dirt on one's shoes, chemical residue on store receipts), choosing safe cookware, reducing the consumption of fish high in mercury, and having clean air in work and home environments (avoiding inhaling particulate matter from industrial exposure, idling trucks, and other vehicles.) Additional measures include choosing products that are heavy metal–free, including personal care products and thermometers, heating/cooling thermostats, and barometers.

When considering a detoxification program, including the removal of mercury-containing fillings, it is important to work with a team of knowledgeable and experienced professionals. Heavy metal exposure may come from a variety of sources, and detoxification requires a systematic approach that may take many months and involve more than one practitioner. When detoxing mercury, lead, and other heavy metals, we recommend educating yourself as much as possible to understand the testing and treatment process.

Foods, Supplements, and Therapies
There is a long list of chelators that may be recommended by practitioners — foods, supplements, and therapies that combine with heavy metals and then carry them out of the body. The list includes:

- Vitamin C
- Chlorella
- Bentonite/fiber (psyllium drink)
- Selenium
- Cilantro
- DMSA
- Bentonite/clay foot or body baths
- Colonics and enemas
- Far-infrared sauna
- Zeolite
- Sulfur-containing foods

Whether to Replace Amalgam Fillings
Some people who have "silver" amalgam fillings containing mercury are able to efficiently eliminate heavy metals from the body on their own, and toxic amounts do not accumulate in the tissues. When there are no noticeable symptoms, however, the only way to know if there has been a toxic buildup in the body is through testing.

Individuals who have "silver" fillings and are concerned about mercury exposure may choose to consider replacing them. Here are some suggestions and considerations:

- Obtain a comprehensive evaluation by both medical and dental practitioners that includes testing.

- Consider working with a trained health coach to integrate lifestyle changes before, during, and after removal. Other pillars of health such as food and nutrition, sleep and breathing, movement and exercise, avoidance of environmental toxins, and loving and nurturing relationships may all play a role in detoxification and improving overall health.
- Every person seeking care is encouraged to become a wise healthcare consumer. Even if there is evidence of heavy metal toxicity, chelation may not be the best first step. It can be expensive, and for patients with other health issues, chelation may be too aggressive.
- Get more information: For resources related to mercury and dentistry, as well as a listing of dentists who are trained in safe amalgam removal, see the International Academy of Oral Medicine and Toxicology at iaomt.org. To find a physician who has training and experience with chelation therapy, visit the American College for Advancement in Medicine (ACAM) at acam.org. There are also functional medicine doctors found at ifm.org and other types of practitioners who do chelation, and it is important to review their websites and speak to the doctor or a representative to familiarize yourself with the process.

Mercury Amalgam Removal Tips
Find a holistic physician to assess and prepare you for mercury amalgam removal and detox.

Ideally, to ensure health and safety while progressing through the mercury detoxing process, have a team in place. A dentist, physician, and health coach trained and experienced in mercury removal should be part of your team. Remember, you are the most important member of the team. Be sure the treatment meets your individual needs, and have your practitioners collaborate with one another. Ask questions and get answers you understand. Make sure to seek information about the following:

- Clearing and strengthening the detox pathway that all heavy metals must use in exiting the body
- Pacing the detox process (including weight loss, if appropriate) so as not to overwhelm the detox pathway
- Designing and helping you follow diet and lifestyle choices that support the entire immune system so the body doesn't succumb to infections and inflammation during the healing process

Removal of mercury amalgam fillings from the mouth — A checklist for patients

Removing mercury from the mouth carries significant hazards if handled improperly, so it is imperative that you find a qualified dentist trained in using mercury-safe techniques to replace or remove the mercury amalgam fillings from your mouth.

When mercury fillings are being replaced or removed, mercury is released at a high rate and the danger of mercury poisoning is the greatest. Some people have become desperately sick because sufficient precautions were not taken. Proper technique is even more important when the fillings also combine mercury, nickel, and/or copper alloys, which exacerbate mercury's toxic effects, and/or the patient carries one or more copies of the ApoE4 gene.

Before scheduling an appointment to have any silver fillings removed, you may want to call the office for answers to the following questions about the dentist's practices:

- *Is this practice both mercury-free and mercury-safe?*
  Mercury-free dentists refrain from placing new mercury fillings. Mercury-safe dentists follow strict protocols when removing mercury fillings to minimize the exposure of mercury vapor to the patient, staff, and environment.

- *What kinds of protective barriers are used in your office during removal of existing mercury fillings?*
  At the very least, doctors should be using the following: Eye protection for the patient and staff, nasal coverage with alternate air supply for the patient, gas masks for the staff, and oversized drapes to cover patients. This is extremely important.

- *Does your doctor use a dental dam during mercury filling removal?*
  The doctor should use a non-latex dental dam to catch any mercury that may fall into the oral cavity. Better still, they should use a suction tip under the dam to pick up mercury vapors. Some mercury-safe dentists prefer to use multiple suction techniques instead of a dental dam, but this is not recommended. Some protective barrier should be in place no matter what.

- *How do you keep from heating up the mercury filling during removal?*
  Copious amounts of cool water should be sprayed on the point of contact of the drill with the filling in addition to the water spray coming from the dental handpiece.

- *How do you protect the room air?*
  During mercury filling removal, two high-volume suctions should be at the site of mercury filling removal to pick up mercury vapors and mercury fillings. Mercury-safe dentists typically have air filters and ion generators in treatment rooms to help with air purification.

- *What kind of filling material compatibility testing do you use, if any?*
  No single dental material is "the best" for every person. Serum compatibility and Meridian Stress Assessment are familiar techniques

used by mercury-safe dentists to select the best materials for each patient.

- *Is a mercury separator installed as part of the office plumbing to prevent mercury pollution of water supplies?*
  Each state has its own regulations governing medical and dental procedures. A mercury separator is a requirement in New York.

- *Does the office use digital X-rays only?*
  You want individual as well as panoramic X-rays to be digital because digital has about 90 percent less radiation exposure. The use of nondigital X-rays could indicate an office uses outdated techniques.

- *How is the mercury filling removed from the tooth?*
  Using new burrs, mercury-safe dentists try to remove mercury fillings in "chunks" to minimize vaporization and tissue contact with mercury material.

- *Is there any special rinsing provided during and after removal?*
  Many mercury-safe dentists use oral rinses before starting removal of mercury fillings and provide multiple rinses during and after the removal procedure. Rinsing with chlorella before and after will absorb escaping mercury.

- *Does the office follow a particular sequence for removing restorations (mercury filling, metal crowns, etc.)?*
  Mercury-safe dentists follow different sequencing strategies, but at this time, no definitive research has proven one is any better than another.

Conclusion

Heavy metals are naturally found in the earth's crust, and the human body uses some of them like copper and zinc to perform its basic functions. However, heavy metals such as mercury and lead can accumulate in the body's tissues and are neurotoxic, impacting the central nervous system and the brain. Over the past century and a half, due to pollution in our environment and a proliferation of chemicals and products containing these metals, including "silver" amalgam fillings, our daily exposure has grown and with it, a buildup of these toxins in the body. Fortunately, we have become aware of this problem and there are different ways to test for these metals and detoxify the body if a person's "body burden" has become too great. Once a person begins exhibiting symptoms of memory loss, heavy metals are certainly one of the important sources to consider.

10

Inflammation and Infections

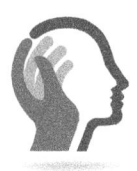

THE BODY'S NATURAL REACTION to a physical injury or insult of almost any kind is to mount a response to minimize the damage. Inflammation is the result of that response, and most of the time, it is felt as pain or heat, or perhaps bloating or other types of discomfort. However, there are times when the body has a reaction and there are no symptoms, although damage is being caused internally. This may be the case with an oral infection or food sensitivity.

Because of the wide range of reactions in the body, it is important to monitor inflammation, as it signifies the body is under stress. Inflammation that does not resolve and remains unchecked can lead to disease and illness, not only in the body but in the brain as well.[400] The most common forms of dementia, Alzheimer's disease, and vascular dementia are associated with a "chronic and exaggerated inflammatory response."[401]

A 2018 study from Johns Hopkins University found that people who experienced chronic inflammation for much of their adult life had more white matter damage in the brain. Since white matter is responsible for transmitting nerve signals, there is a high correlation between chronic inflammation and dementia.[402]

Inflammation may be caused by pathogens (bacterial, viral, fungal, parasitic, etc.), irritants, injury, or oxidative stress. Sources of these effects may be heavy metals, chemicals, and infections. Other potential causes of inflammation include food sensitivities and allergies; prescription drugs and over-the-counter medications; stress, sleep, and breathing problems; and trauma.

In this chapter, we will discuss inflammation and how it is measured. We will talk about infections and low-grade conditions that cause inflammation that often go undetected and yet can cause serious damage to the body and the brain. While any foreign "invader" will cause inflammation, some low-level infections are often overlooked and may be more common as we age. Problems with memory may stem from underlying inflammation. For this reason, it is imperative that testing be done to determine the root cause of the inflammation. It is these types of conditions that can often cause a misdiagnosis of dementia or Alzheimer's disease.

Detecting Inflammation in the Body

When the body is experiencing inflammation from an acute source such as a bee sting or a laceration, the area may be red, swollen, hot, and sore. By comparison, longer-term, systemic inflammation develops over months or years and may not be detected as quickly. Signs of this type of inflammation include skin rashes, excess mucus production, fatigue, and problems with digestion.

A commonly recognized blood test to detect inflammation is high-sensitivity C-reactive protein (hs-CRP). A CRP level between 1 and 3 milligrams per liter of blood (mg/L) often signals a low, yet chronic, level of inflammation. A result above 3 mg/L denotes a high risk for heart problems. There is a strong relationship between the health of the heart and that of the brain. Levels above 10 mg/L may indicate impaired immune response or inflammatory disease.[403] The erythrocyte sedimentation rate is another blood test used for people with inflammatory conditions such as rheumatoid arthritis.

Doctors also measure homocysteine levels to evaluate chronic inflammation. Homocysteine is a type of amino acid that the body uses to make proteins. Elevated levels of homocysteine in the blood can reveal a vitamin deficiency (B6, B12, or folic acid) or may indicate heart disease. The normal range of homocysteine is less than 15 micromoles per liter (mcmol/L); high levels point to inflammation in the body. Another test physicians use is HbA1c — a measurement of blood sugar — to assess possible damage to red blood cells.

Elevated white blood cell count (WBC) is a way to measure infection, a more acute form of inflammation. White blood cell count rises as the body mounts an immune response. When the situation resolves quickly, the site of the infection begins to heal. It is when white blood cell counts remain high that there is an indication something else might be going on such as infection, stress, inflammation, trauma, allergy, or certain diseases. That is why an elevated WBC count usually requires further investigation.

For individuals who carry at least one copy of the ApoE4 gene, a full discussion of biomarkers that may be important in detecting inflammation can be found at ApoE4.info/wiki/Biomarkers.

Inflammation can be caused by any number of exposures and insults to the body and, if left untreated, lead to dementia. When the infection or inflammation site is known, the symptoms can be seen as described above. But when inflammation is asymptomatic, it may go undetected for a long time. For that reason, testing is the primary way to identify if there is a systemic problem. Addressing the causes of inflammation, discussed next, as early as possible will prevent further damage to the body. A healthy diet that contains anti-inflammatory foods and avoids inflammatory foods, maintenance of normal blood sugar, exercise, and stress management all aid the body in reducing inflammation.

Food Sensitivities

The health of the gut microbiome is a relatively new area of study in the medical literature. Its importance has grown as we have come to understand that a healthy gut reflects the strength of the immune system. Caring for our gut flora starts in utero as nutrients are shared between mother and fetus. Vaginal births enrich the gut microbiota and hence the immune system of the newborn; the high incidence of Cesarean births in the United States poses a disadvantage for the immune system of these babies when compared to those coming into the world via natural birth.[404]

Gut flora that is not sufficiently populated with a diversity of organisms has been thought to lead to some childhood diseases and conditions, including autism and ADHD.[405, 406] The underdeveloped immune system, perhaps further disadvantaged by a diet of man-made formula and foods containing chemicals and GMOs, may not be able to support the schedule of immunizations that babies receive in those first years. It is not the vaccines themselves, perhaps, but the condition of the host that is the issue.

From birth, our diets play a role in our overall health and well-being. A poor diet without enough nutrients can break down the digestive tract and its thin cellular wall, leading to a condition known as "leaky gut."[407] Leaky gut occurs when the cell wall of the intestines becomes permeable and food particles get through this natural barrier and enter the bloodstream. A standard American diet (SAD) high in processed foods that contain an abundance of simple carbohydrates and sugar, coupled with a stressful life, is often responsible for many of the digestive ailments and symptoms doctors are seeing:

- Acid reflux, heartburn, and gastroesophageal reflux disease (GERD)
- Irritable bowel syndrome (IBS)
- Crohn's disease
- Dyspepsia/indigestion

- Nausea and vomiting
- Peptic ulcer disease
- Abdominal pain syndrome
- Belching, bloating, and flatulence
- Biliary tract disorders, gallbladder disorders, and gallstone pancreatitis

If the root causes of digestive ailments, including leaky gut, are not known or addressed, inflammation can create one or more of these conditions in the gut and cause damage throughout the body.

Testing for Food Sensitivities
There are a number of ways to test for food sensitivities, but the most common is a blood test that measures the body's immune response to certain foods. A test that measures the body's immediate autoimmune response after eating a particular food is called an IgE test (immunoglobulin E) and is the one many doctors use to detect a food allergy. Symptoms might include a rash, hives or itching, anaphylaxis, and swelling of the mucous membranes.

An IgG (immunoglobulin G) blood test detects subtler responses to foods that can emerge up to three days after the food is consumed. Foods with high IgG scores are considered food intolerances. Symptoms typically are more systemic in nature and cause chronic inflammation. Many of these are unfortunately common ailments today and include constipation, Crohn's disease, diarrhea, eczema, flatulence IBS, migraines, obesity, and psoriasis.

In addition to blood tests, another way to determine sensitivity to foods is an elimination diet that omits foods that may be causing intestinal discomfort. Such common allergens are dairy products, gluten, eggs, shellfish, and nuts; these and other foods may be eliminated for two to three weeks and then, one at a time, added back into the diet to see how well they are tolerated. There are many types of elimination diets, and they typically take several weeks to complete. Working with a doctor or health coach will ensure that the diet and reintroduction of foods provides the most accurate results.

Another type of diagnostic test for the gut microbiome is a stool analysis. Some companies offer at-home test kits where a sample is submitted to a laboratory and the patient receives the results via email. These tests vary in the information they provide and cost. Most tests analyze the microorganisms in the patient's gut; require a survey about lifestyle, metabolism, diet, and genetics in order to produce a profile; and then make suggestions for improving the microbiome. Many integrative doctors use stool tests as part of their comprehensive evaluation of health and to determine whether the gut microbiome has a good balance of beneficial and harmful bacteria.

Treating Food Sensitivities
Once food sensitivities and intolerances have been identified, the foods are removed from the diet for a period of time and then can be reintroduced. Through this process, much of what has been causing the discomfort should ease. After inflammation is reduced, symptoms have abated, and the gut has healed, continuing to eat a healthy diet is key. Our bodies function well when we eat whole foods that our bodies easily recognize and process. When we eat "junk" foods, and "food-like" substances that are created in a laboratory and have little nutritional value, our digestion continues to suffer.

A digestive tract's "good bacteria" thrive on fibrous foods that contain inulin, fructo-oligosaccharides (FOS), and galacto-oligosaccharides (GOS), known as prebiotics. Some examples are garlic, onions, leeks, chicory root, dandelion greens, Jerusalem artichoke, asparagus, bananas, and some grains such as oatmeal and barley.

Probiotics help the microbiome stay in balance and are considered "good" bacteria. Typically fermented, probiotics are found in foods such as kimchi, sauerkraut, pickles, miso, tempeh, and kombucha.

Yogurt and a similar food, kefir, are known to contain healthy quantities of probiotics. Common probiotic strains are lactobacillus, bifidobacterium, and saccharomyces boulardii and can be helpful for different intestinal conditions.

Working with someone who can help identify the cause(s) of intestinal problems and the source of inflammation, and then provide guidance on diet and dietary habits, will often heal the distress. This may include an integrative or functional medicine doctor, a gastrointestinal (GI) specialist, and/or a health coach.

Preventing Food Sensitivities
What one eats, the way the food is grown and prepared, and a person's eating habits all contribute to good health. Foods may have been sprayed with chemicals, grown with pesticide and herbicide applications, injected with hormones, or be laden with preservatives, artificial flavors, and colors. Another consideration is the environment in which we eat. Do we sit down relaxed and in good company, starting the digestive process by eating slowly and chewing the food? Or are meals eaten while watching TV or doing other tasks, so that eating is a means to an end? All of these considerations impact digestion and gut health.

Food sensitivities may have a genetic component, but eating a diet rich in whole foods and drinking pure, uncontaminated (filtered) water is a good first step in avoiding food sensitivities. Fruits and vegetables are best washed before consuming, and buying animal protein where the animals are raised in humane conditions and are grass-fed provides the cleanest food options and will help to minimize inflammation.

Lyme Disease

Lyme disease was reportedly first detected in Lyme, Connecticut, in the late 1970s when a group of adults and children was afflicted by arthritis-like symptoms. The disease was traced to a deer tick that transferred a bacterium called *Borrelia burgdorferi* to humans in the form of a spirochete, which can be difficult to track in the human body. Although some scientists believe the bacterium to be much older, it is the transference to humans and the long-term ill effects that make it so problematic today.

If a tick bite is noticed quickly and a diagnosis is made, Lyme disease can often be treated and cured with oral antibiotics. If, however, the disease is not detected or diagnosed and symptoms begin to worsen, it is often much more difficult to treat both the disease and its symptoms, some of which persist for a long time, if not indefinitely. In addition, the disease can lead to a host of medical, neurological, and psychological conditions as it disrupts the immune system and causes the type of systemic inflammation that leads to memory loss.

According to the CDC, Lyme disease symptoms include a "'bull's eye' rash, fever, chills, headache, fatigue, and muscle and joint aches; swollen lymph nodes may occur in the absence of rash. Longer-term effects may include severe headaches and neck stiffness; additional rashes on other areas of the body; facial palsy (loss of muscle tone or droop on one or both sides of the face); arthritis with severe joint pain and swelling; intermittent pain in tendons, muscles, joints, and bones; heart palpitations or an irregular heartbeat; episodes of dizziness or shortness of breath; inflammation of the brain and spinal cord; nerve pain; and shooting pains, numbness, or tingling in the hands or feet."[408] Most importantly for our discussion, 70 percent of people with Lyme disease report changes in their thinking such as memory loss and reduced mental sharpness,[409] and this can happen at any age. Neurological symptoms include:

- Impaired attention, focus, concentration, judgment, and impulse control
- Impaired memory and speech functions
- Disorganization and loss of direction

- Poor problem-solving and decision-making abilities
- Slower mental processing speed

Lyme Disease Prevention, Testing, and Treatment
As with many other diseases, prevention of Lyme disease is key. When spending time outside in an area where deer populate, or if hiking or walking in the woods, it is essential to wear long pants and shirts with long sleeves. Applying essential oils that repel insects or using other natural insect repellents is helpful. Afterward, a thorough inspection of the body will detect any ticks; many people do not feel it when they are bitten. Ticks must be removed carefully with tweezers and clothes washed and dried (a clothes dryer will kill deer ticks). Monitor the site carefully, be aware of any symptoms, and if they appear, be sure to get treated within three weeks to minimize long-term effects. Unfortunately, blood testing in the first several weeks can show false negatives because of the time it takes for antibodies to develop, so many doctors prescribe antibiotics prophylactically.

The CDC recommends a two-step testing process: A sensitive enzyme immunoassay (EIA) or immunofluorescent assay (IFA) followed by a Western immunoblot.[410] Both are required and can be done using the same blood sample. If the first test is negative, no further testing is recommended. If the first test is positive or indeterminate (sometimes called "equivocal"), the second test should be performed. The overall result is positive only when the first test is positive (or equivocal) and the second test is positive (or for some tests, equivocal).

If you think you have been bitten by a tick or exhibit symptoms described above, your doctor will prescribe a course of antibiotics. After that, a holistic approach to reduce inflammation, enhance lymphatic and liver activity, boost the immune response, and restore gut homeostasis will likely be effective. Make sure to seek out practitioners who have experience and success with treating Lyme disease.

Mold Exposure

People have varying sensitivities to mold, which are multicellular organisms that can exist in our environment and go undetected. Mold typically grows in places that have too much water or dampness and that do not have a chance to dry out. Whether in the home or office environment, mold illness can trigger a host of chronic health problems. Because mold is becoming a more prevalent issue across the United States often due to violent rainstorms, flooding, and homes that are many decades old, studies are looking at its effects on the human body. These effects include:
- Brain inflammation in the hippocampus, the area of the brain that governs memory, learning, and the sleep-wake cycle
- Decreased neurogenesis, or the formation of new brain cells
- Impaired memory
- Increased sensitivity to pain
- Increased anxiety[411]

Many people are familiar with mold spores, but the spores are not always responsible for mold toxicity. Molds produce mycotoxins, toxins that are small enough to pass through most materials, and they trigger an immune response that can cause symptoms and illness like those above through inflammatory effects. Children, due to their size, are more susceptible to the adverse effects of mold.

There are many types of mold, and the type can determine how mold is treated and remediated. Common molds include aspergillus, Cladosporium, and stachybotrys atra (also known as black mold). Aspergillus is a type of mold often found on foods and in home air conditioning systems and can cause allergic symptoms. Stachybotrys is one of the most dangerous types of mold and can cause flu-like symptoms, diarrhea, headaches, memory loss, and severe respiratory damage.

Chaetomium is another common mold found in homes with water damage. Able to thrive in wet, dark environments such as drywall, wallpaper, baseboards, and carpets, Chaetomium is similar to black mold. It might cause general signs of allergies such as red, watery eyes and trouble breathing, as well as neurological damage and certain autoimmune diseases.

Acremonium is a type of mold which starts off as moisture in small areas and leaves a powdery substance that may be pink, gray, orange, or white. Acremonium is dangerous and can grow alongside other molds. Health problems that result from exposure include autoimmune and bone marrow disease.

Molds such as aspergillus and penicillium can be found in the air and become problematic with overexposure, often in confined environments. These molds cause breathing problems, bronchitis, and other infections. Another mold called alternaria can be airborne in warmer months.

These are just some examples of molds that can cause toxicity and a host of health issues. If you smell or see mold, make sure to investigate and have the problem addressed.

Symptoms of Mold Exposure

People who have had exposure to indoor mold often exhibit upper respiratory tract symptoms that include, but are not limited to, coughing, sneezing, and wheezing; itchy eyes, nose, and throat; runny or stuffy nose; postnasal drip; dry, scaly skin; and restricted breathing and other airway symptoms. More research needs to be done to determine the longer-term effects of mold exposure. Depending on the type of mold, other symptoms might include aches and pains, changes in mood, headaches, memory loss, and nosebleeds.

Mold Testing and Treatment

An initial and easy test for mold exposure is an online visual contrast sensitivity test. It is considered nonspecific and will show a deficit for people who have been exposed to biologically produced toxins. Occupational exposure to heavy metals, solvents, petrochemicals, and hydrocarbons are all known to create deficits in visual contrast. A test that measures visual contrast sensitivity can be taken online at VCSTest.com and will help to confirm whether there is a problem.

If you think you have been exposed to toxic mold at your home or office and want details about the specific mycotoxins, at-home tests can identify the type of mold in your environment and determine whether it is toxic. Environmental relative moldiness index (ERMI) or health effects roster of type-specific formers of mycotoxins and inflammagens (HERTSMI) tests can identify whether there is a mold problem, and sampling is done from floor dust where mold spores are most likely to be found. Air testing is also used. Knowing the type of mold will then help to dictate the best course of action and treatment. If the testing is positive, it is critical to take action to remediate the situation. ERMI and HERTSMI tests are available in a test kit or from companies that do mold testing.

You may want to seek professional help to confirm test results and have the area in question remediated. Environmental mold testing requires a thorough visual inspection for any water damage or mold growth and an air quality test to check for airborne spores. Samples are sent to an independent environmental testing lab to determine whether harmful mold spores are present. Mold remediation specialists can remove the toxic mold in your home and evaluate any remaining sources of water damage. Once the mold has been remediated, a clearance air test can be performed to ensure that mold levels are safe and in the normal range.

Mold does not go away on its own, and, if left untreated in the body, can create serious physical problems, causing inflammation and affecting memory. If you see or smell mold or start to feel unwell inside a building, remove yourself from the area.

Oral Infections

Many people have heard of systemic infections, such as Lyme and other tick-borne diseases, and problems associated with exposure to mold toxins. Less well known, and often undetected, are the kinds of infections that begin in the mouth and can metastasize systemically and impact brain health. Oral infections progress from the oral cavity to secondary systemic effects via three mechanisms or pathways:

- Metastatic spread of infection as a result of transient bacteremia
- Metastatic injury from the effects of circulating oral microbial toxins
- Metastatic inflammation caused by immunological injury induced by oral microorganisms[412]

Low-level infections in the mouth fall into two main categories: periodontal disease and endodontic disease.[413]

Oral Infections — Periodontal Diseases

Periodontal diseases are complex, chronic, infectious, and inflammatory conditions of the gums and other tissues supporting the teeth. The bone around the teeth deteriorates, and as that happens, gum pockets develop in the spaces that open up, and bacteria begin to populate those pockets. The bacteria/disease weakens the bone and other tissues supporting the teeth, and eventually, those tissues lose their ability to hold the teeth. As the protective barriers normally provided by healthy gum tissue break down in the mouth, inflammation and the invasion of bacteria into the blood system follows, resulting in systemic interactions such as metabolic syndrome,[414, 415] obesity,[416, 417] diabetes,[418, 419] stroke,[420, 421] osteoporosis,[422, 423] and autoimmune disorders.[424]

It is also now widely recognized that the inflammation associated with periodontal disease is also associated with a higher risk of cardiovascular disease and diabetes as a result of the elevation of specific inflammatory proteins that can be measured in the blood. One of these compounds, C-reactive protein, is now recognized as a stronger predictor of an initial cardiovascular event than LDL cholesterol levels.

In addition, evidence suggests periodontal disease may also be responsible for brain dysfunction. Pathogens associated with periodontal disease have been found within the blood vessels that communicate with the brain, suggesting they migrate to the brain from the oral cavity through the vascular system. This may compromise blood flow to the brain and introduce pathogens and their toxic waste products into the brain.

Along the same lines, a study by the University of Central Lancashire (UCLan) School of Medicine and Dentistry suggests "people with poor oral hygiene or gum disease may be at a greater risk of developing Alzheimer's disease." In brain samples donated by ten patients without dementia and ten patients suffering with dementia, the researchers detected the presence of Porphyromonas gingivalis, a pathogenic bacterium, in the brains of patients with dementia. This same group, in collaboration with the University of Florida, used animal models to confirm that P. gingivalis in the mouth often finds its way to the brain once periodontal disease has set in.[425]

A 2023 review and meta-analysis of studies that looked at the connection between oral bacteria and dementia showed a ten- and sixfold increased risk of AD when there were oral bacteria and Porphyromonas gingivalis, respectively, in the brain.[426]

According to the U.S. Surgeon General's report, most adults show signs of periodontal or gingival diseases. Severe periodontal disease (measured as 6 millimeters of periodontal attachment loss) affects about 14 percent of adults aged 45 to 54.[427] In addition, 23 percent of 65- to 74-year-olds have a severe periodontal disease.[428] At all ages, severe periodontal disease is more likely to be found among men, people at the lowest socioeconomic levels, and smokers.[429]

Treating Periodontal Disease

Diagnosis of periodontal disease is based on a clinical examination, and new methods are evolving for DNA testing of the pathogens present in a given patient. Controlling the plaque and the body's reaction to it is key to getting the problem under control, but sometimes that is much easier said than done, especially if a local infection has metastasized into the bloodstream and has become systemic. In such cases, systemic inflammation exacerbates the reaction of the gums to the plaque that is building up around the teeth. Although most dentists view dental disease as having a local cause rather than a nutritional one, systemic infection is far easier to eradicate when treatment includes correcting the patient's body chemistry, including saliva pH, calcium, phosphorus, and intake of refined carbohydrates. Since humans are physical as well as energetic beings, the overall energetic state of the individual is also important to consider. If the patient is symptomatic, the problem may be treated homeopathically or through other means.

Treating periodontal disease involves cleaning accumulated biofilm or plaque off the teeth and then educating the patient on how to use home care methods to keep plaque from rebuilding on the teeth and reversing the development of gum pockets created by the deterioration of the bone around the teeth.

Treatment options have improved over time. In the past, the only way to clear plaque and bacteria was to cut away gum tissue to reduce the depth of the pocket, making it easier to reach the plaque building up on the teeth. Now, due to advances in technology, dentists have much less invasive and less extreme methods for even advanced gum disease, such as using lasers that allow for the correction of gum pockets without cutting away the gums. This is a gentle therapy that promotes reattachment of the gums to the root surface.

There are other measures that are especially useful for aged patients who are experiencing signs of dementia. These patients may lack the manual dexterity or mental focus to use home care methods effectively. Using a water irrigation device such as a water flosser can help, though sometimes it is not enough. Often a medication known as Arestin (low-dose doxycycline) will be placed into infected pockets to block the proliferation of bacteria.

Other Interventions
To reduce the need for surgery for patients with serious periodontal disease who have difficulty getting their plaque under control, an alternate treatment method[430] can be highly effective: A small amount of a peroxide gel is placed in a custom-fitted tray and worn for 10 minutes at a time a few times during the day. This cleans out bacteria so the body has a chance to heal.

Essential Oils
Because antibiotics and other treatments for periodontal disease can cause side effects, there is a need for alternative approaches. Essential oils, which are distilled from plants, have been used for centuries in various cultures. The quality of the oil is important, and only pure essential oils should be used for medicinal purposes. These oils are so potent that they often must be diluted before they can be applied, but this does not alter their anti-bacterial, -fungal, and -microbial properties. A study that reviewed clinical research and relevant articles concluded that essential oils have the potential to be developed as preventive or therapeutic agents for various oral diseases, although more research needs to be done.[431]

Another study that used various essential oils showed that those with antibacterial properties could be effective against oral pathogens that contribute to infection. Peppermint, tea tree, and thyme oil can act as an effective intracanal antiseptic solution against oral pathogens.[432]

In clinical practice, other essential oils with some of the properties noted above have been used for particular conditions. These include clove oil, myrrh, spearmint, and eucalyptus. For patients experiencing chronic periodontitis, the combination of essential oil mouth rinse and subgingival ultrasonic instrumentation has been shown to reduce bacteria in both shallow and deep pockets.[433] A holistic dentist may be able to guide patients on the use of essential oils to manage symptoms and healing of oral infections and gum disease.

In some cases, salt water rinses with or without baking soda, hydrogen peroxide rinses, and cold compresses can help with symptoms as well.

Oral Infections — Endodontic Diseases

Endodontic diseases share several similarities with periodontal disease: Both are complex, chronic infections that cause inflammation. However, while periodontal disease affects the gums and teeth, endodontic disease starts in the soft tissue inside the tooth (the pulp) and can spread to the areas around the tooth root. From there, it can affect other parts of the body.

The spread of infection from endodontic disease can lead to systemic health issues as bacteria and toxins enter the bloodstream. Additionally, infections in the teeth may affect the body through the autonomic nervous system, which can be evaluated by holistic dentists trained in specific techniques such as applied kinesiology.

Bacteria from infected teeth pose similar risks to those seen in gum disease. Endodontic disease may result from bacteria entering the pulp tissue, repeated trauma to a tooth, or even complications from root canal treatments.[434] Since performing a root canal treatment can sometimes introduce bacteria into the bloodstream, it is essential to maintain good oral health through proper diet, oral hygiene, and preventive care. A balanced diet that limits sugars and fermentable carbohydrates — such as those found in grains and sweets — is critical, as these foods encourage the growth of bacteria responsible for tooth decay. Diets high in fermentable carbohydrates can also lead to changes in gut health, encouraging the growth of harmful fungi.

Diagnosis and Testing

Low-level chronic infections of the teeth may be difficult to detect. There will not always be pain present.

Oftentimes X-rays show evidence of a deteriorating root canal treatment. This would typically be evidenced by a deficient seal of the root canal at time of prior treatment. With conventional 2D X-rays, we may see evidence of pathology in the bone around the tooth as a result of chronic persistent infection. With the advent of the 3D cone beam X-ray, pathology related to an infected and/or root canal–treated tooth can be more accurately diagnosed.

Both muscle-response testing (kinesiology) and electroacupuncture diagnosis will provide evidence of the systemic ramifications of a diseased tooth.

Treating Endodontic Disease

Numerous treatments can be considered, but for a patient with debilitated health and an infected toxic tooth, very often the best choice is to remove the tooth. It is important that the infected area around the tooth be thoroughly cleaned to remove residual infection. In addition to physically scraping the bone, it is advisable to flush with sterile saline and infuse the bone with ozone gas if available to further reduce the potential of residual microorganisms.

Responsible Use of Antibiotics and Protecting Your Gut Flora

Infections treated with antibiotics wipe out both bad and good bacteria in the gut microbiome. Many holistic dentists avoid prescribing an antibiotic to reduce risk of postoperative infection because it may induce resistant bacterial strains and disrupt gut ecology. Herbal formulas are an alternative. Individuals should work with their doctor to replace the good bacteria and provide supplementation, if necessary, following a course of antibiotics. Examples of prebiotics and probiotics are previously noted in the Food Sensitivities section.

Preventing Oral Infections

Preventing periodontal disease is entirely possible with attention to dental hygiene, healthy diet, and physical exercise. Individual nutritional and lifestyle habits greatly influence who is at risk for gum disease, who actually gets it, how it starts, and what events occur as the disease progresses, both locally in the mouth and throughout the body. According to the research being amassed, diet and nutrition are key. Many of the dietary suggestions found in the Nutrition and Supplements chapter of this book apply here, and some specific supplements are discussed below.

The Role of Diet and Nutrition

The foundation of a healthy immune system is always a fresh, clean diet with plenty of organic fruits and vegetables plus daily exercise. If the food we eat now were as rich in minerals, enzymes, vitamins, microbes, and other nutrients as it was 100 years ago, taking supplements would probably not be necessary.[435] However, the soil is so depleted of nutrients today[436] that such supplementation can produce important benefits. A study conducted by researchers at Loma Linda University showed that a nutritional supplement alone (from Pharmaden Nutraceuticals), without any other dental treatment, was able to significantly mitigate the effects of periodontal disease, lowering bleeding and reducing pocket depths.[437] Ingredients in the supplement included CoQ10 (ubiquinone), vitamin C, echinacea, folate, and grape seed extract. While vitamin D was not part of the Pharmaden study, it is a critically important nutrient for dental health; many people are deficient in vitamin D, especially during colder months when they do not spend as much time outside.

Taking adequate quantities of the following five supplements can help to prevent periodontal disease in the first place, aid in healing, and prevent the disease from recurring.

- **CoQ10 (ubiquinone).** CoQ10 improves the body's overall healing response. It is vital to all natural processes including the production of cellular energy, immune system function, heart function, and blood pressure. It has been studied for use in the treatment of congestive heart failure, neurodegenerative disorders such as Parkinson's disease, and cancerous tumors. *Special warning for those on statin medication:* Individuals taking statins for cholesterol management should consider taking a CoQ10 supplement, since statins can dangerously lower the body's production of CoQ10.

- **Vitamin D.** Periodontal disease often leads to tooth detachment due to acid leaching of calcium. Research shows that this condition causes chronic inflammation and is linked to low serum 25-hydroxyvitamin D (calcidiol) levels.[438]

- **Folic acid.** Folic acid is required to ensure normal development of gum tissue. It binds to and neutralizes the bacterial by-products known as endotoxins.

- **Echinacea.** Echinacea is a very powerful herb that has been used as a home remedy for colds and the flu. For treating periodontal disease, it inhibits enzymes that break down tissue.

- **Grape seed extract (GSE).** Case study reviews in Italy and France have found measurable health benefits from certain compounds in red grapes called proanthocyanidins,[439, 440] which have 20 to 50 times the antioxidant power of vitamin C or vitamin E. They are also a natural antihistamine and able to counteract allergies without causing drowsiness, natural anti-inflammatories useful against arthritis and CRP, beneficial for skin problems, and supportive of the circulatory system. In its particular application to periodontal treatment, GSE prevents bacteria from colonizing in the gum tissues and on the teeth and blocks the aggression of destructive enzymes. GSE's antioxidant action also destroys free radicals that attack the gum tissue.[441]

The Role of Exercise

Diet and exercise can reduce gum disease by 40 percent, according to researchers from the Case Western Reserve University who examined data from 12,110 individuals.[442] They found that those who exercised, followed healthy eating patterns, and maintained a normal weight were 40 percent less likely to develop periodontitis. They also found that periodontitis was reduced by 29 percent for those individuals who met only two of the healthy behaviors and 16 percent in those that met at least one.

The researchers concluded that healthy behaviors such as exercise and diet that lower the risks of diabetes can also lower the risk factors for periodontitis. Exercise is known to reduce the C-reactive protein in the blood, which is associated with inflammation in the heart and periodontal disease. Healthy eating habits, which build the body's defenses against disease, also reduce the production of plaque biofilm, which is the primary epidemiological factor associated with periodontal disease.

Urinary Tract Infections

Urinary tract infections (UTIs) are not uncommon in older adults, and they can go undetected if a person is asymptomatic. UTIs account for about 25 percent of all infections of the elderly, especially those in nursing homes.[443] Any infection in the body can cause inflammation, and if the infection remains unchecked, it can lead to systemic inflammation that affects the brain. In older people with memory issues, a UTI is often accompanied by confusion and sometimes delirium. This is because the brain becomes inflamed and cognition is impaired. For individuals who regularly suffer from UTIs, it makes sense to have a doctor test them periodically and try to address the underlying cause.

Other Ways to Treat Systemic Inflammation

In this chapter and in much of this book, we have talked about the most common sources of systemic inflammation and how each of those causes can be identified, addressed, and prevented. Here are a few other suggestions that might be helpful to discuss with your doctor.

Reducing Inflammation in the Body

As mentioned previously, the body mounts an immune response to any pathogen, injury, or condition it feels needs to be managed or contained. This chapter has addressed some of the causes of inflammation that lead to memory problems; however, systemic inflammation from almost any cause can lead to inflammation of the brain. Some examples are autoimmune diseases, smoking, obesity, alcohol, and chronic stress.

What can someone do to lower inflammation in the body? The suggestions cover a wide range of options including diet, exercise, herbs, and pharmaceutical medications. For example, certain foods are known to be pro-inflammatory or anti-inflammatory:[444]

Foods That Promote Inflammation
Refined carbohydrates such as sugar, white bread, and pastries
Fried foods such as French fries
Red meat
Processed meats such as hot dogs and sausage
Dairy products
Nightshade vegetables (peppers, eggplant, white potatoes, and tomatoes)

Foods That Lower Inflammation
Olive oil
Leafy greens such as kale and spinach

Fatty fish such as salmon, mackerel, anchovies, sardines, and herring
Nuts and seeds
Fruits, especially cherries, blueberries, and oranges
Water/adequate hydration

Some herbs and spices have an ameliorative effect on inflammation and are listed below. As always, individuals should consult their doctor before taking any supplements.

Turmeric (Curcuma longa) is a spice popular in Indian cuisine that has been used since ancient times and contains over 300 active compounds. The main active component is an antioxidant called curcumin, which has powerful anti-inflammatory properties. Curcumin is found in the turmeric root; it blocks inflammatory cytokines and enzymes in two inflammatory pathways. Several human trials have shown an anti-inflammatory benefit,[445] which can translate to reduced joint pain and swelling. Other anti-inflammatory herbs are black pepper, bacopa monnieri, lemon balm, rosemary, ginkgo biloba, gotu kola, sage, ashwagandha, ginseng, cinnamon, nutmeg, mint, saffron, and thyme.[446]

Finally, inflammation sometimes can be reduced by using ice and/or heat. Ice typically is used on acute injuries within 48 hours to lessen swelling and reduce inflammation. Heat is often used for chronic conditions to stimulate blood flow and ease achiness of muscles and tissues. Epsom salts baths are another way to ease pain and reduce inflammation.

Conclusion

Inflammation, often due to infections in the body, is a fact of life that results from interacting with our environment. Inflammation can have many sources and may or may not produce symptoms. For example, some people experience digestive discomfort over a period of time and never suspect that they may have leaky gut. Alternatively, if someone has recently had oral surgery, this may account for some residual pain. If the reason for the inflammation does not resolve on its own, seeing a doctor is a logical next step. Inflammation markers in the blood will certainly help to determine if there is an issue. Where memory loss and dementia is concerned, undetected infections and sources of inflammation can be a critical underlying factor to understanding the disease and need to be evaluated and treated.

11

Prescription Medication

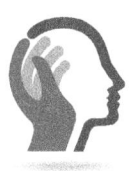

PRESCRIPTION DRUGS CAN BE LIFESAVING and life prolonging, and yet almost all are known to have at least some side effects. When patients are prescribed several different medications by different physicians and experience new symptoms, it can be hard to know whether symptoms reflect the disease, side effects from the medication, or the interaction between the various drugs. The first order of the day is to make sure patients are given only the medications they require and only for as long as is necessary. If an individual shows signs of cognitive impairment, examining the person's prescriptions is vital in eliminating what might be a reversible cause of memory loss and dementia.

It is not uncommon to hear stories about "miraculous" cognitive recovery taking place when patients discontinue a recently prescribed medication. Often the patient's cognition is rescued by an advocate, a family member, or a friend who insists that doctors or hospitals discontinue a medication that isn't proven to have a specific lifesaving or pain-controlling purpose. One renowned integrative clinic made it a practice for each patient to bring every medication, supplement, and over-the-counter remedy they were taking into the clinic and provide the frequency, dosage, and length of time they had been taking each one. This is good practice, as it ensures that those caring for the patient are aware of their entire regimen.

This chapter will cover a general approach to working with your doctor and then explore the most common drugs that affect, or have side effects that interfere with, healthy brain function.

Working With Your Doctor on New Medications

Many medications and supplements may directly or indirectly impact cognitive health. Specific drugs are addressed in the next section. The Sharp Again Medical Advisory Board supports a cautious approach when adding new medications. Many drugs provide significant benefits but are often prescribed to treat symptoms without addressing the root cause of the problem or without full consideration of potential side effects. For this reason, it is recommended that everyone work with their doctors to minimize the use of unnecessary medications. Here are a few questions to ask when discussing a potential new drug:

- *What is the root cause of the condition or symptoms that the medication is treating, and does the new medication address what is causing the problem? If not, is there a way to treat the underlying cause?*
  It is common for medications to treat symptoms without addressing the root causes. Treating symptoms may be the best science has to offer, but it is important to learn whether the cause of your symptoms has been identified and can be treated.

- *Can I effectively treat this problem by making lifestyle changes instead of starting a new medication?*
  This will vary, based on the individual's condition or disease, how acute it is, and whether lifestyle changes can be sustained. Making changes to one's lifestyle to solve a health issue is preferable since it more often addresses the root causes and avoids potential adverse side effects from medication.

- *How long will I need to be on this medication? What changes do we need to see for me to end the drug eventually?*
  When starting a new medication, it is useful to set the criteria for ultimately moving off the drug. In some cases, this may include specific lab test criteria or the implementation of lifestyle changes that lead to measurable results. Some medicines may need to be used indefinitely; however, by working with your doctor to see if there are other ways to improve your health over the long term, you may be able to take a lower dosage or potentially transition off the medication.

- *Does this medication have any possible interactions with the medicines or supplements I am currently taking?*
  Everyone's physician and pharmacist should routinely be checking for potential drug interactions. However, they may not know all the medications, over-the-counter supplements, or remedies you regularly use. Asking this question ensures that nothing is overlooked.

These recommendations should not create the impression that medication is harmful because many drugs provide significant health benefits. However, it is not unreasonable to question the typical approach of solving a health problem with a pill when there may be effective ways to address the same problem without the harmful side effects. Asking our doctors questions and advocating for ourselves and our loved ones will help to ensure everyone receives the care they need.

Medications Known to Compromise Cognitive Function

Prescription and nonprescription medications that increase the risk of dementia fall into three primary categories: anticholinergics, benzodiazepines, and statins. Each type of drug has a different relationship to cognitive health and is explored below.

Anticholinergics
Anticholinergics block the action of the neurotransmitter acetylcholine. Found in the central nervous system, the visceral motor system's ganglia, and neuromuscular junctions, the blockage of acetylcholine increases the risk of dementia.[447] Of primary concern are the vast number of medications that have anticholinergic properties. They are prescribed or available over the counter for conditions affecting all of our organ systems. These medications may be quite beneficial individually, but at higher doses, with prolonged usage, and in combination with others, unwanted side effects become more likely.

Most Common Side Effects of Anticholinergic Medications
- Confusion, disorientation, and memory problems
- Headache
- Dry mouth and nose
- Decreased sweating
- Dizziness, drowsiness, and unsteady gait
- Constipation
- Difficulty urinating
- Visual difficulties

Anticholinergic medications can provoke a less common but far more severe set of side effects: an acute confusional state where the patient is disoriented and may act bizarrely. When blood levels of the medication recede, the confusion might end, leaving the person with no recall of the episode (and which they may vehemently deny has occurred). In response, a physician might put the patient on medications to control what seems to be a "psychosis"; however, when combined in the aggregate, some of these medications can have enough anticholinergic effects of their own to be fatal.

Anticholinergics encompass a broad class of medications, which includes the following drug categories:

Categories of Anticholinergics
- Antihistamines — allergy treatments, nighttime pain relievers
- Antidepressants — mood and neuropathy (nerve pain) medications
- Incontinence and overactive bladder (OAB) medications
- Antidiarrheal medications
- Anti–motion sickness medication
- Anti-dizziness medications
- Some asthma medications
- Antianxiety medications
- Acid-blocking ulcer medications

Benzodiazepines

Benzodiazepines are a category of medications used to reduce anxiety, promote sleep, and relax muscles. They adversely affect cognitive function, so much so that long-term use is explicitly described as elevating the risk of developing Alzheimer's disease.[448]

When stress is expressed as anxiety and difficulty sleeping, many people turn to pharmaceuticals such as benzodiazepines. A study conducted by researchers from France and Canada found that the widely prescribed benzodiazepines are associated with an increased risk of developing AD. The researchers found that the higher the dosage and length of the patient's use of benzodiazepines, the greater the risk of developing AD. Risks were highest for people who frequently used higher doses of benzodiazepines for five years or more. Compared to individuals who took no sleep medication whatsoever, patients who took the equivalent of full daily doses for three to six months over a five-year period were 32 percent more likely to develop AD. The risk factor rose sharply to 84 percent for participants who had taken a benzodiazepine for over six months.[449, 450] Fortunately, there are safer options for those experiencing difficulty sleeping (see the Sleep and Breathing chapter).

Here are commonly prescribed benzodiazepines:
- Alprazolam (Xanax)
- Chlordiazepoxide (Librium)
- Clonazepam (Klonopin)
- Clorazepate (Tranxene)
- Diazepam (Valium)
- Lorazepam (Ativan)
- Triazolam (Halcion)
- Zolpidem (Ambien)
- Eszopiclone (Lunesta)
- Zaleplon (Sonata)

Statins, used to lower cholesterol, are the most widely prescribed medications in the world. Brand and generic names include:
- Altocor
- Atorvastatin
- Crestor
- Fluvastatin
- Lovastatin
- Lescol
- Lipex
- Lipitor
- Lipostat
- Livalo
- Mevacor
- Mevastatin
- Pitava
- Pitavastatin
- Pravachol
- Pravastatin
- Rosuvastatin
- Selektine
- Simvastatin
- Torvast
- Zocor

Cholesterol is a complicated subject that is also discussed in depth in the Hormones chapter. Meta-analyses present conflicting data on the role of cholesterol in the body and specifically in the brain. These analyses suggest that our genetic profile, age, and gender are factors to consider in the decision to take a statin. High cholesterol in midlife has been associated with an increased risk in Alzheimer's disease and vascular dementia.[451] For that reason, if someone has a genetic predisposition for high cholesterol and heart disease, doctors will likely prescribe a statin to protect vascular health. It is recommended that patients also be informed of lifestyle changes that can positively impact cholesterol prior to, or coupled with, a statin prescription.

In the context of brain health, the definition of a high cholesterol level is more nuanced. Many doctors consider a total cholesterol level of 190 high enough to recommend statins, as "normal" ranges have been lowered in recent years. However, research indicates that cognitive impairment is also common at cholesterol levels below 200.[452] This finding is not surprising, since the brain is the most cholesterol-dense part of the body, harboring 20 percent of all its cholesterol.[453] Defects in brain cholesterol metabolism have been shown to be implicated in neurodegenerative diseases such as AD.[454] This is a viable concern, and each patient must consult with their doctor to determine the best course of action.

In later life, cholesterol likely has a protective effect on the brain, especially for women.[455] One study showed that higher levels of HDL cholesterol positively correlated with better cognitive function in adults over age 60.[456] An article in *Experimental Gerontology* states: "Randomized controlled trials and most longitudinal observational studies do not show a positive effect of statin treatment on the risk of dementia when prescribed in later life."[457] In fact, studies show that the inverse may be true.[458] While there is evidence to suggest that statins can have a protective effect on the brain, other data indicate some statins can be harmful to the brain, liver, and muscles.[459, 460]

One of the mechanisms by which statins may interfere with cognition is by inhibiting the synthesis of Coenzyme Q10. CoQ10 is an extremely important carrier and transmitter of the energy produced in the mitochondria, as the cells metabolize glucose to generate the energy needed for all of life's processes. That energy is stored in a molecule that gets created called adenosine triphosphate (ATP). When the statins decrease the synthesis of CoQ10, not enough ATP is produced. This impacts the organs in the body, including the brain, and memory and cognition can decline. Statins can also interfere with ATP production in the muscles, resulting in muscle pain and weakness. Because of this impact on the body's CoQ10, many in the medical community have recommended CoQ10 supplementation to their patients.

The understanding of statins and, more generally, of cholesterol and lipids is continuing to evolve. While it is clear that statins can be a valuable tool for cholesterol management, as with any medication, they may also produce unwanted side effects and risks. It is worth exploring lifestyle approaches to control cholesterol and lipids through diet and exercise. There are very different and complex opinions on the subject, so individuals should discuss their specific situation with their doctor.

Coming Off Medications Safely

CAUTION: Under no circumstances should individuals take themselves off prescription medication without a medical doctor's guidance and instructions for doing it safely.

Most physicians have more experience putting patients on medications than taking them off those same medications. Patients often have to advocate for reduced dosing or ceasing medications, and individuals may choose to initiate a conversation with their doctor if they are experiencing side effects or feel the medication is no longer effective or necessary.

Mood and Pain Medication

Healthcare providers generally agree that medications designed to manage mood and pain should be withdrawn gradually, not only to prevent physical and emotional distress but also to give the individual a chance to determine how well they adapt to the withdrawal of chemical support. A strong social network and access to professional support can be important in dealing with the withdrawal effects of medication.

The question of addiction is becoming better understood, and more doctors are aware of the need to support patients desiring to get off medications. Rehabilitation might be an essential part of helping a patient reduce dependence on certain drugs.

Statins

Individuals should consult their healthcare provider when trying to reduce or eliminate statins. A doctor may suggest lowering the dosage or combining the medication with another drug. Gradually tapering off a cholesterol medication, especially from higher dosages, is advisable to allow the body to adjust and to reduce the risk of a serious heart event.

Conclusion

It is important for everyone to know why a medication is prescribed and to consider whether the intended results might also be achieved by employing nonpharmacological approaches. For example, if someone is showing a fasting glucose in the prediabetic or diabetic range, instead of choosing medication as the first step, a possible initial approach would be to address nutrition and lifestyle factors. Eating a healthy diet by reducing refined carbohydrates and sugar, getting adequate exercise and sleep, and addressing stress might very well have a positive impact on insulin resistance and reduce or eliminate the need for medication.

If medication is necessary, individuals should make their doctors aware that they want to be on the medication for as short a time as possible to achieve the desired results. As with any new medication, it is important to make sure doctors are also aware of all the other prescription medications and supplements patients are taking.

12

Physical and Emotional Trauma

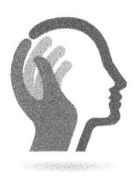

TRAUMATIC EVENTS IN OUR LIVES — from verbal, physical, and emotional abuse to accidents, brain injury, and PTSD — can all contribute to future cognitive dysfunction. Recent research suggests that both physical and emotional trauma may increase the risk of developing dementia later in life.[461] As previously discussed, chronic stress that may result from trauma leads to elevated cortisol levels, which have been linked to the shrinking of brain regions involved in memory and cognition, such as the hippocampus. Emotional trauma, including unresolved grief, anxiety, and depression, can further accelerate cognitive decline by disrupting neural pathways and increasing inflammation in the brain.[462] Adverse childhood experiences (ACEs), such as abuse, neglect, and household dysfunction, are particularly impactful, as early-life trauma can result in long-term changes to brain structure and function, weakening cognitive resilience over time. Furthermore, physical injuries, especially traumatic brain injuries (TBIs), may hasten the onset of neurodegenerative diseases such as Alzheimer's.[463]

As our understanding of the link between the mind and body grows, it is clear that trauma — whether physical or emotional — can have lasting effects on memory and brain health. Addressing all types of trauma is critical to reducing the risk of future cognitive decline and preserving long-term brain function. In this chapter, we discuss the types of trauma, what causes them, how they impact the brain, and how to treat them.

Traumatic Brain Injury (TBI)

A single trauma to the brain may cause changes in brain tissue that may eventually lead to neurological diseases such as Parkinson's and Alzheimer's. The older one's age when experiencing a TBI, the higher the likelihood that memory loss will accompany the injury.[464]

When the skull is hit hard (referred to as blunt force trauma, e.g., from a fall or from a blow to the head), a series of events takes place. For a fraction of a second, millions of minuscule bubbles will form in the solid matter of the brain and will then quickly dissipate. However, a swath of destruction is left in the wake of this swarm of nanobubbles. Specifically, the bubbles trigger the release of glutamate, a neurotransmitter that, when released in excessive amounts, acts like shrapnel on nearby neurons (a process called "neurotoxicity").

In the case of a concussive injury, it is the neurometabolic disturbance in the brain which leads to the challenges with brain function. Whatever the mechanism by which the physical trauma works, there are downstream consequences that manifest themselves in pathologies, typically a disruption of anatomical structures, a disruption of function, or both. Some of these pathologies are of academic interest only, due to the fact that they don't (yet) translate into something that can be easily addressed and remedied. However, there are other pathologies that offer hints about steps that can be taken to improve recovery and restore function.

One of the important pathologies of TBI and of Alzheimer's disease is that neurons become starved for fuel — that fuel being glucose. There is no shortage of glucose or insulin in the body; these are in abundance. Rather, the trauma to the brain disrupts the insulin receptors on the neurons so that these receptors can no longer activate a portal (think of it as a turnstile) that is needed to transport glucose into the cell.[465] It is similar to plugging up a car's gas tank with rags — the fuel can't get in. With little or no glucose getting in, these neurons falter. The clinical result is slow thinking, difficulty taking initiative, problems following through, dysregulation of affect, and the like. In other words, all the major aspects of executive function have been diminished.[466]

General Symptoms of Traumatic Brain Injury

Even though a loss of consciousness is a good indicator of a concussion or TBI, there are many other milder symptoms that should be cause for concern as indicators of a concussion.

Most people are familiar with the physical symptoms of a concussion — headache, sensitivity to light or noise, fatigue, blurry vision, balance problems, nausea, or fatigue. But there may also be cognitive issues such as having difficulty concentrating or remembering new information, becoming easily fatigued by reading or using a technological device, or not being able to process things as quickly.

There can be disturbances in sleep such as an increased need for sleep or restless sleep and/or difficulty falling asleep. Finally, mood issues can also be a symptom of a concussion, including anxiety, agitation, irritation, sadness, and emotional volatility. Symptoms vary from person to person depending on the area of the brain affected as well as the severity of the concussion.

Long-Term Effects of Traumatic Brain Injury

Ten to twenty percent or more of patients who experience a concussion go on to develop chronic issues as a result of head trauma, called post-concussion syndrome, in which symptoms persist for longer than six weeks. In some cases, symptoms can persist for weeks, months, or even years.[467]

The more head injuries a person has, the greater the chance of developing post-concussion syndrome, and the damage can accumulate with repeated injury. This long-lasting inflammation can result in greater activation of the stress response cycle, impairment of gastric motility, and compromise of the immune barriers of the intestines and the brain. It may even result in emotional dysregulation or in debilitating sensory disturbances such as the inability to tolerate loud places or busy visual patterns. Some people may also develop learning difficulties, personality changes, and other cognitive deficits. Any number of neurological symptoms may become permanent as well, including loss of taste or smell, ringing in the ears, motion sickness, or mood disorders.

Treatment of Traumatic Brain Injury
Treatment for TBI will vary based on the severity of the injuries, and for most accidents, it is important to seek medical help immediately. Although the body is designed to heal itself, the central nervous system cannot resolve inflammation as easily as the rest of the body. Once there is inflammation in the brain, it tends to remain for quite some time, delaying the healing process. The inflammation and symptoms of a concussion can continue after the initial injury for months or even years without proper treatment.

A traditional medical approach for treating TBI includes acute care, surgery, rehabilitation (including physical and occupational therapy), cognitive behavioral counseling, and other interventions.

Integrative therapies known to help TBI and restore brain function include neurofeedback and hyperbaric oxygen therapy (HBOT).[468, 469] Acupuncture, cranial sacral therapy, meditation, and energy work have been used clinically, but no empirical studies have been conducted. Examples of other potentially useful treatments include balance therapy, vision therapy, and neuro-optometric rehabilitation. The goal is to avoid medications whenever possible since the system is more sensitive to these after a brain injury. In the case of a severe concussion or TBI, it may be necessary to use anti-seizure medications for a short period of time. What follows is some information on other treatments that may be useful.

Ketones
As noted earlier, in Alzheimer's disease, as with TBI, there is a very similar disruption of the insulin receptors on neurons. This is why both conditions respond so well to foods and "medical foods" that provide ketones, such as coconut oil and its derivative, MCT oil.

Ketones are the final breakdown product of fat metabolism. When you ingest coconut oil, the liver converts it into "ketone bodies" that passively diffuse into the neurons (no receptor needed, no turnstile involved). These ketones thereby provide an "alternative fuel" for the brain. The brain is thus a hybrid engine. If it cannot get glucose, it can utilize ketones. This has been important for species survival in periods of famine: The body will break fat down into ketones that keep humans alive in the face of starvation. Functional and integrative practitioners in clinical practice have seen coconut oil produce significant gains in people with dementia, TBI, and Parkinson's disease.[470,471]

Some physicians have been skeptical about the potential benefits of coconut oil, which may stem from a lack of awareness of the metabolic strategy underlying its usage. Numerous scholarly articles have been published on the subject, and one of the most compelling facts is that, gram for gram (actually, mole per mole), each molecule of ketone produces vastly more energy (as a high-energy molecule called ATP) than does each molecule of glucose.[472] Coconut oil is also discussed in the Nutrition and Supplements chapter.

Side effects of coconut oil include loosening of stools and even frank diarrhea. For anyone contemplating using coconut oil, it is prudent to start with a low dose, e.g., ¼ teaspoon once per day, and build slowly, perhaps to one full tablespoon twice a day. Note that administering coconut oil, MCT oil, or other ketone strategies to someone who has dementia might cause them to suddenly become much more active.

They can injure themselves because they do not have full awareness. It is advisable to "safety-proof" their living space to prevent injuries.

Omega 3s

There are several natural treatments for a concussion that assist with decreasing inflammation in the central nervous system, thereby allowing healing to proceed faster. These include high doses of good quality fish oils to help improve blood flow to the brain as well as provide the building blocks for healing cells of the central nervous system. Omega 3 supplements are usually sourced from the tissues of oily fish, such as salmon, tuna, herring, mackerel, or krill. Some studies have also used plant-based oil supplements. Quality is important because some fish oils are tainted with mercury, PCBs, and other toxins.

Rest and Gentle Exercise

Rest immediately following a concussion for a day or two is important and includes additional sleep as well as limiting screen time from phones, computers, and television exposure. Once it has been determined that there is no structural damage to the brain such as bleeding, rest needs to be paired with gentle activity to encourage good blood flow to the brain and stimulation of different brain areas to support healing. Gentle exercise that does not risk re-injury such as walking or rhythmic movements can be very helpful. A stationary bicycle and swimming can also be excellent forms of gentle exercise that increase blood flow and coordination.

Additional Supplements to Consider

Micronized progesterone (a bioidentical form) and small doses of lithium orotate can help decrease the exaggerated inflammatory response in the brain.[473, 474] N-acetyl cysteine may also be helpful for many people to decrease overstimulation of the brain. Overall, a person's nutrient status should be optimized, especially for levels of magnesium, zinc, copper, B vitamins, vitamin D3, and antioxidants.

Other Treatment Options

Many of the medications and nutraceuticals that help patients who have dementia are also helpful for patients who have TBI. A compilation of useful ideas for treating TBI can be found in the *Textbook of Traumatic Brain Injury*.[475]

Prescription Medications
In the *Textbook of Traumatic Brain Injury*, the "Psychopharmacology" chapter lists medications that can be useful in treating the cognitive impairments seen in TBI, including stimulants (methylphenidate and dextroamphetamine), amantadine, bromocriptine, Sinemet (levodopa/carbidopa), modafinil, and donepezil. These may be worth considering, particularly if the nutraceuticals discussed in the next section do not work sufficiently well. Individuals will want to consult with their integrative or primary doctor before starting any prescription medication.

Nutraceuticals
Another helpful chapter in the *Textbook of Traumatic Brain Injury* is "Alternative Treatments" by Dr. Richard Brown and Dr. Patricia Gerbarg. In the chapter, the authors list a number of nutraceuticals with which they have reported positive clinical outcomes. These include acetyl-L-carnitine, citicoline, S-adenosylmethionine (SAMe), B vitamins, and others.

It is worthwhile to know about these, that they are available, and that they can work for many people. For those who have suffered a TBI, it is advisable to consult integrative psychiatrists and other physicians familiar with supplementation.

Hyperbaric Oxygen
Hyperbaric oxygen treatment can be very helpful for the treatment of concussion and TBI[476] because it supports the energy centers of the

cell, which accelerates healing. Acupuncture has also been shown to be helpful for mobilizing energy to accelerate healing of concussions and decrease pain.

Neurofeedback (NF)

NF is a type of biofeedback where the "signal" to be trained is the amount of abnormal neuronal activity in various regions of the brain. Some regions are underactive, which can be seen on a computer-based analysis of brain activity called a quantitative EEG (qEEG). These underactive regions can be "tuned up" through biofeedback.[477] For example, when the underactive region in question happens to show more activity, the individual is "rewarded" by being able to continue watching a chosen video. The video will stop running if the individual slips out of that zone of activity. The cumulative effect of this training (over many sessions) is a meaningful improvement in executive function.

Yoga

Unfortunately, people with TBI can come to hate their brains, and hate themselves, which sends them into a vicious downward spiral. Practicing yoga can help in several ways. It connects a person more fully to their body, experiencing a connection with breath that helps the body find a way to "live" with the disability that has been suffered. Yoga teaches individuals to be less judgmental and more accepting of the limitations they might be experiencing.[478, 479] Yoga also stimulates the autonomic nervous system and tones the vagus nerve, which may help with recovery by building resilience.[480]

Preventing Traumatic Brain Injury

Many suggestions about preventing TBI may seem obvious, but people often are in a hurry or forget to pay attention to the small things that can have profound consequences.

- Try to avoid all trauma to the head. Group sports begin at relatively young ages and are often played throughout life. It is not uncommon for children to get hit in the head with a ball or experience some type of head trauma from falling off a bike or when skating or skiing. While one hopes that children are resilient and recover, it is now known that these events may have a cost, especially if sports are played through high school and into adulthood. There are many well-documented cases of professional football and soccer players developing chronic traumatic encephalopathy (CTE) and Alzheimer's disease. Adults and children should take proper precautions when engaging in sports that involve frequent falls. If a concussion does occur, seek medical attention immediately.
- Fasten your seat belt. Most auto accidents occur within a mile or so of the home. One does not have to go through the window to suffer a devastating TBI. Just a solid tap of the head against the glass or steering wheel, at a decent speed, can cause lifelong injury.
- Make a mental note when overhanging objects are there. If you are about to bend down under an open cupboard door or underneath a stairwell, remind yourself of the danger before doing it. Otherwise, when you absent-mindedly stand back up, you will get a whack.
- Don't put objects down in the path where you or others will be walking. Instead, put things down along the wall or in a corner.
- "Watch where you're going" is a common admonishment. Perhaps a better phrase would be "Go where you're watching." If you can't see the path clearly, don't go. It could be that the path (e.g., through a room) is dark, that you're carrying objects that partially obscure your field of vision, or that you're looking at your cell phone or tablet as you walk. Whether the ensuing fall smashes your head or fractures your hip, it's a chance you don't want to take.
- Be mindful and observant for other potential hazards: cracks in the sidewalk, sidewalks pushed up by the roots of a tree, rough patches of pavement, and of course, icy patches (especially on grates and on those metal gates that open to store basements).

- Never walk with your hands in your pockets. If you trip and cannot get your hands out to break your fall, you can experience a life-altering injury.
- Take classes to improve balance. These include yoga, Tai Chi, Qigong, and balance classes at the Y, the health club, or at a local medical center. These classes can prevent falls and can teach skills to land more safely if you do fall.

Emotional Trauma

Trauma can be defined as an event which overwhelms the nervous system, something very distressing or upsetting, and in which a person feels helpless (witnessing or experiencing something horrific, where they fear that they or someone else is at risk of injury or death). Trauma that lasts many months or years, and that goes untreated, can damage the physical, emotional, and mental health of an individual at any stage of life. Even single traumas left untreated can leave a permanent imprint upon the nervous system.

Such varied experiences may include the destruction of prized possessions, loss of freedoms, or lack of safety or security. Most frequently, traumatic experiences are connected to abuse, abandonment, or neglect and may be physical or emotional in nature.

Almost any experience can cause trauma to develop when a person's unique ability to cope is exceeded. Feeling helpless in the presence of a stressor and unable to deal with the situation can determine whether an event is experienced psychologically or physiologically as trauma.

Emotional trauma may be experienced at any age. Research shows that early childhood adversity, sometimes referred to as adverse childhood experiences (ACEs), can impact memory function later on in life. When researchers looked at traumatic events experienced by children, those who reported having at least one ACE (and for many children, there were multiple) had a greater likelihood of cognitive dysfunction in midlife and a higher incidence of dementia in later life.[481]

Physiological Changes Caused by Emotional Trauma
Trauma changes the brain and its chemistry and can cause epigenetic changes (the interaction of genes and the environment) that can be passed onto the next generation, even during pregnancy and in infancy.[482, 483] Most importantly, trauma can have a lasting impact upon the nervous system, and trauma "memories" become a burden to the body by over-activating or under-activating the autonomic nervous system. Some people who have experienced trauma endure prolonged periods of arousal or agitation followed by mental, emotional, and/or physical exhaustion and burnout. Reactions to trauma are usually an unconscious process, and during periods of reactivity, memory skills can falter and it can become difficult to perform even simple cognitive tasks.

Stress experienced from a traumatic event or series of events causes an increase in levels of adrenaline and cortisol, two stress hormones tied to survival. Chronically high levels of stress, especially combined with conditions that threaten our physical and psychological well-being (toxic stress), result in sustained and elevated stress hormones. This cortisol "bath" often leads to adrenal fatigue, insomnia or hypersomnia, learning difficulties, poor memory, and difficulty making decisions.

Post-Traumatic Stress Disorder (PTSD)
Post-traumatic stress disorder is included in the *Diagnostic and Statistical Manual of Mental Disorders* (DSM-5) as a Trauma- and Stressor-Related Disorder and is no longer considered an Anxiety Disorder. PTSD can happen after a deeply threatening or fear-inducing event. The aftermath may involve reliving the event or forgetting part or all of it. There are numerous criteria highlighted in the DSM-5 that need to be met, and PTSD is often misdiagnosed.

Research shows that veterans with PTSD have a higher likelihood of developing dementia, and it is not uncommon for their PTSD symptoms to last years or decades if left untreated.[484] To complicate matters, those with PTSD often have suffered a traumatic brain injury (TBI), which would further increase the chance of developing dementia.

Individuals who experience emotional trauma in childhood have a higher likelihood of developing PTSD.[485] Even if trauma is experienced as an adult, the risk of developing dementia increases.[486] In another study, those with PTSD had twice the incidences of dementia than their non-PTSD counterparts.[487] People with PTSD are also more likely to experience depression, which is highly correlated with dementia.[488] Research shows that not only can prolonged sadness create inflammation in the body, depression also is associated with a reduction in cerebral blood flow, which is known to precede cognitive decline.[489] While depression can often be treated, in an elderly person suffering from dementia, the treatments have not been shown to be effective and may actually cause harm, resulting in falls, hospitalizations, and a higher risk of mortality.[490] Additionally, recent research shows there is potentially an additive effect of depression and chronic stress for those suffering from PTSD, increasing the risk of mild cognitive impairment and Alzheimer's disease.[491]

PTSD is best addressed by a professional with specialized training, due to the wide range of treatments and therapies that are available. If someone has experienced trauma of any kind, professional help is usually required. Like most of the causes of dementia, the sooner treatment is sought, the higher the likelihood that memory issues can be prevented, arrested, or at the very least, delayed.

Adverse Childhood Experiences (ACEs)
Adverse childhood experiences (ACEs) are experiences that happen when we are young, and these experiences can have a profound impact on memory, health, and well-being later in life. These early life experiences include physical, mental, emotional, sexual abuse, and/or neglect; abandonment; malnutrition; poverty; and other traumas (additional types include fires, severe weather events, accidents, severe medical interventions, war, death, and domestic violence).

A long-term study begun in 1995 by Kaiser Permanente, the Centers for Disease Control, and other institutions[492] looked at the effects of ACEs on health outcomes over time and found strong relationships between ACEs and numerous health, social, emotional, and behavioral problems, including suicide and depression.

The body and the brain are impacted by these adverse experiences. Those who have experienced ACEs often have impaired immune systems where the body's ability to fight disease and infection is compromised.[493] ACEs also affect the structural and functional development of the brain's neural networks, and these changes can impact memory in middle age and lead to dementia later in life. Long-term effects may include premature aging and less resilience in fighting disease.[494]

Children who experience extensive maltreatment have been shown to have smaller brain volume and lower IQ scores, possibly setting them up for neurological disadvantages later in life.[495] Overcoming the effects of ACEs often depends on utilizing a number of strategies that have been proven to promote good health — such as exercising and abstaining from smoking — as well as access to emotional support, building resilience, and having a sense of purpose. The more strategies employed, the better the outcome.

ACEs can cause a cascade of chronic stress reactions and trauma responses. Many therapists are specially trained to treat people who have experienced childhood trauma. Complex post-traumatic stress disorder (C-PTSD), a relatively new category of PTSD, tends to develop as a response to prolonged and repeated trauma, which can be physical, psychological, or sexual in nature. It is a series of emotional "hits" to the nervous system that can lead to dissociation, somatization (physically expressing stress and emotions), and people not having a core sense of who they are.

Symptoms of Emotional Trauma
Trauma can be experienced emotionally, cognitively, and physically.

The severity of symptoms in response to trauma depends on the individual, the type of trauma, and other factors. If an individual has experienced trauma, they may display immediate or delayed symptoms and behaviors including but not limited to:
- Intrusive and recurring thoughts or memories with an inability to push them out of the mind for very long
- Flashbacks ranging from brief distractions to a loss of awareness and feelings of disorientation
- Detachment from the self and others, such as an inability to express emotions, lack of empathy, or avoiding or being unable to form connections on an emotional level
- Recurrent nightmares or night terrors
- Re-experiencing or the sense of reliving past event(s), including body sensations
- Difficulty integrating and/or making sense of what has happened
- Struggling to cope
- Intense feelings of anger, sadness, and fears that are inappropriate, incongruent, or disproportionate to current events
- Anxiety/panic disorders and/or various mood disorders/depression, especially if the person does not respond well to medications or traditional talk therapies
- Hypervigilance with difficulty or an inability to relax or let down one's guard
- Feeling insecure, unsafe, and unable to trust others
- Difficulty establishing or maintaining healthy, loving, safe, and respectful relationships
- Feelings of low self-esteem, lack of self-worth, and poor boundaries

Following a traumatic episode, a racing pulse, nausea, chronic pain, and muscle tightness can persist or reappear suddenly at inappropriate times long after the environmental trigger for a "flight-or-fight" response is gone. Research shows that trauma affects the whole body — disrupting the immune, endocrine, and muscle systems and setting the stage for diseases such as immune and autoimmune conditions, chronic pain, substance abuse, anger and fear issues, and a host of other medical conditions.[496]

With unresolved traumas, emotions can swing rapidly and become intense and overwhelming. If feeling afraid, angry, or out of control, traumatized individuals may withdraw, cutting off those closest to them. When someone is emotionally distressed, cognition is impaired, and this may negatively affect memory or attention.

Our thinking may be affected by a persistent "brain fog" or problems with focus and attention, and we may develop cognitive challenges. We might become easily distracted, struggle to concentrate on tasks that once interested us, and have difficulty remembering things. We might even forget the events surrounding the trauma, as these memories become inaccessible to our consciousness. Alternatively, when the trauma stays with us, C-PTSD symptoms can arise, including aggressive, emotional outbursts, sleep disruption, self-destructive behaviors, chronic illnesses, and feelings of alienation or dissociation.[497]

The emotional and cognitive effects of trauma are well known and widely discussed in the media in connection with veterans returning from combat. However, we often neglect to acknowledge and properly address the toll of less severe traumas on our bodies and minds. For example, children who are repeatedly humiliated or criticized or who are raised with stress and a feeling of helplessness can experience trauma. Whether mild or pervasive, unresolved trauma is stored in the body and in the brain.

Although the traumatic event may be long over, someone who is traumatized may continue to experience memories of it, along with a physiological stress response. Our brains and bodies get amped up, ready to respond to the trauma-inducing stressor, and the body cannot return to equilibrium. Without help, the body cannot complete the response needed to escape from, fight against, or otherwise resolve the trauma. Traumatic memories might "loop" as cognitive patterns and affect the neurologic circuitry of the brain.

Treating Emotional Trauma
Leading researchers and clinicians in the field of trauma research recognize that trauma and stress are stored in the body — literally in the cells — and not just in the brain. The body is always sending sensory and perceptual messages to the brain, and it is important to pay attention to those cues.[498]

Many of us are familiar with therapies in which patients explore childhood experiences and talk extensively with a therapist, seeking the situational roots of their traumas and any emotional or cognitive symptoms they may be experiencing.

Some clinicians who treat trauma suggest that another way of dealing with unresolved traumas may be to focus on the physiological experience — delving deep into what they describe as the "traumatic energy" stored in our bodies. It is through somatic experience — that is, working with the body — that emotional trauma can be fully released.

Contemporary trauma experts Dr. Bessel Van der Kolk and Dr. Peter Levine have developed highly effective therapeutic approaches to trauma resolution that address the physiological roots of the stress response. In their approach, talk therapies and pharmacologic interventions alone do not go deep enough to get to trauma's root cause, which is often in physiological and psychological response patterns. When patients talk about their unresolved traumatic memories, the emotional part of the brain becomes triggered, the patient becomes hyper-aroused and may physiologically feel flooded with emotions again, and the cycle continues. This is why they recommend a slow and paced approach to treatment.

Body-Focused Trauma Recovery

To understand how the key to trauma recovery may lie in "letting our bodies speak," it is important to first understand the body's physiological response to stress. How do wild animals deal with threats? Animals facing serious, life-threatening danger have three instinctive defense systems for dealing with the threat:

- They can develop sudden tonic immobility where muscles go limp and they are frozen and unable to move.
- They can go into fight-or-flight-or-freeze mode. The sympathetic nervous system pumps out many neurochemicals or hormones readying the animal to attack or flee, and in some cases, mammals are known to "freeze" or shut down bodily responses in order to feign death.
- They can seek social engagement to defuse tension and reduce the threat. Animals are wired to seek safety in numbers and find comfort with others. This support-seeking behavior only occurs in mammals.

Humans share similar survival instincts. When confronted with overwhelming or life-endangering stress, we respond like threatened animals, and we cannot talk or reason ourselves out of these instinctual, physiological, and largely unconscious responses.

Dr. Peter Levine developed an approach to treating trauma called Somatic Experiencing (SE) to help patients tap into the body's natural release and reset mechanisms. Somatic or body-focused approaches to trauma recovery acknowledge the mind-body connection. They are designed to recruit the body to work with the brain to release and then integrate mental and sensory memories from the past. Somatic therapies help trauma sufferers pay attention to and observe physical sensations as a means of accessing and releasing stored energy from unresolved trauma.[499]

SE is based on the natural mechanisms wild animals use to restore their physiological equilibrium after stressful events. Animals have been observed to shake their bodies involuntarily to release stress chemicals and excess energy. Humans sometimes find themselves shaking uncontrollably after stress, but in modern society, we have been conditioned to suppress this natural stress response. We may also be distracted from allowing ourselves to "shake off" trauma when forced to deal with the immediate aftermath of traumatic experiences.[500]

Somatic-based therapy practitioners use techniques that allow clients to slowly and safely release the "stuck" energies that are held in their bodies and that are negatively affecting their lives. Through body-aware psychotherapies, clients can allow the energy to release little by little in a controlled environment by crying, shaking, or experiencing other modes of gradual and gentle release. Without addressing these locked-down energies, trauma can be continually re-experienced through physical sensations and emotions that arise even without conscious awareness or direct memories of the trauma. Dr. Francine Shapiro and Dr. David Grand developed Eye Movement Desensitization and Reprocessing (EMDR) and Brainspotting, respectively. These are both eye-movement and alternating-stimulation techniques which help unlock and resolve stored trauma through sensory and perceptual awareness linked with eye movement or eye position. Both of these methods can be effective alternatives to drug treatment and talk therapies alone.[501, 502]

Acknowledging that trauma is actually "stored" in the body empowers individuals to access professional treatment in the same way they would for any physical symptom or injury that needs time and attention to heal.

Restorative Yoga
There is evidence to suggest that gentle restorative yoga can reduce stress, aid in recovery from trauma, and support brain health. One of the benefits of restorative yoga is that it provides the opportunity

to connect deeply into the nervous system and release tension caused by trauma. It allows people to connect with the internal experience their body is having (interoception)[503] and with the messages they are receiving from their nervous system (neuroception). The practice consists of poses (asanas) that are performed seated, lying, or standing. These postures are held for a period of time to allow a relaxation or deepening into the pose. One of the reasons yoga is beneficial for nervous system and brain health is that the parasympathetic nervous system benefits alongside the vagus nerve. When we engage in many types of yoga positions and include conscious breathing and vocalizing sounds like mantras, we stimulate the vagus nerve, which directly benefits the autonomic nervous system.

It is best to use an integrative approach to healing trauma that includes body movements with one or more of the healing modalities mentioned above. All of these approaches will help with relieving stress and supporting brain health.

Conclusion

Both physical and emotional trauma affect the body and the brain in ways we are beginning to more fully understand. Unresolved emotional trauma and untreated physical trauma at any point in the human life cycle can be a causal factor of dementia. Addressing past traumas can favorably impact our brain health, and those who have suffered traumatic experiences may be helped by an array of interventions and treatments. For that reason, it is critical that medical and lay communities become more aware of this important relationship and encourage patients and loved ones to get prompt treatment.

PART THREE

DON'T WAIT — ACT TODAY!

IT IS HUMAN NATURE NOT TO TAKE ACTION until something is staring us squarely in the face. For over 100 years, we knew about a disease called Alzheimer's, named after the French doctor, Alois Alzheimer, who first diagnosed it but could do nothing about it. As people approached older age, some got this dreaded disease, and others did not. No one knew why, and people were afraid, especially if they had lost a family member to the disease.

In the past 20 years, we have come to understand this disease much better. There are now tests that tell us a decade before symptoms occur whether we have the biomarkers that will likely result in Alzheimer's if we make no changes to our lifestyle. We are beginning to have the information that will motivate us to take action and do what we know is possible to avoid losing our memories.

Unfortunately, our medical system has been slow to catch up with the approaches presented in this book. Neurologists are still diagnosing people with Alzheimer's disease and other forms of dementia and telling them to go home and get their affairs in order. And yet, we know people are getting their minds back day by day, and others are preventing the disease or significantly delaying it, even those with a genetic predisposition.

There is real hope, and Sharp Again will continue to educate people about the causes of memory loss and provide the tools they need to get on a path to better brain health. We will continue to provide resources and coaching to facilitate making changes *today* that will improve not only brain health but overall health and well-being. We will go into underserved communities who rely primarily on family and friends for caregiving to educate and try to stem the tide of dementia. We will continue to monitor research and share with the public what else may be impacting cognition and steps we can take to address these risk factors.

If this book has been helpful to you, we invite you to visit our website, sharpagain.org, and sign up to receive information or make a donation to help support our efforts. Let us know if you would like us to come and make a presentation for your group or do a webinar. Write to us at MYM@sharpagain.org with reviews, a referral to a doctor in your area, or if we can join you in your efforts to fight dementia. We believe everyone deserves to live a long, healthy life with their minds intact. Please help us make Alzheimer's only a memory.

13

Finding Qualified Healthcare Professionals

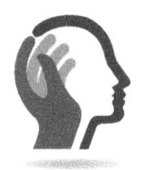

WHILE MANY HEALTHCARE PROVIDERS may be qualified to treat one or more causes of dementia, a functional medicine, integrative, holistic, or naturopathic doctor can often identify the underlying causes of memory loss by looking at the body as a whole and how effectively each system is functioning on its own and in relation to the entire body.

Most traditionally educated medical doctors (MDs) and dentists (DDSs and DMDs) in the United States have not received in-depth training for most causes of memory loss. Medical and dental schools typically do not offer extensive coursework on topics such as nutrition, heavy metals, environmental toxins, stress management, or sleep and breathing issues. For this reason, you may need to go outside of traditional healthcare to find alternative or integrative physicians.

There are a variety of ways to find a practitioner who understands a multi-therapeutic approach to healing, and these are listed next. Many of these doctors partner with health coaches to help patients follow recommended changes to diet and lifestyle, which is useful for prevention as well as following a treatment protocol. Each individual seeking treatment will have their own insurance and financial considerations, and making a decision about which practitioner to use will likely require time and research.

How to Find a Practitioner

Options Available for Finding a Practitioner:
Seek a practitioner recommendation in your area from a trusted friend, colleague, or other medical provider.
Depending on where you live, you may have access to one or more functional medicine or integrative practitioners. If you have friends who have been to integrative doctors, ask for a recommendation. Not all practitioners are aware of the causes of dementia, even though many of them are trained to treat them. As you go about your research, here are some helpful tips:
- Thoroughly read each doctor's website and any printed materials.
- Call the doctor or office manager with questions about their services, policies, practices, insurance, and costs. Some doctors take insurance, and others do not. Depending on where you live and the type of practitioner you are seeking, you may have a wide choice or a very limited one.
- To determine if you've found the right professional, schedule an initial consultation (in-person or videoconference) to see if they are the right doctor for you or your loved one. You want to work with someone who will answer your questions and who treats you with consideration and respect.

Do a Search for an Integrative Doctor or Holistic Dentist
The following websites provide ways to search for doctors in your area:
- IFM.org (Institute for Functional Medicine)
- AIHM.org (Academy of Integrative Health and Medicine)
- IAOMT.org (The International Academy of Oral Medicine and Toxicology)
- Functionalsource.com

In the absence of a trusted personal referral, the next best sources of information on integrative practitioners are websites of the associations to which they belong. Each website has an interactive database that lists member physicians and where they practice. Simply enter your zip code and the number of miles you are willing to travel from your home, and they will tell you which of their members practice in the area.

We suggest you visit several association websites, as it is impossible just from a listing to tell whether a particular physician is right for you. Then, visit websites for the individual doctors to learn more about their qualifications and specialties. You may also want to search sites such as healthgrades.com and vitals.com for reviews.

If you have questions about the practice or services that are offered, call the office and speak to someone.

Find a Health Coach to Support You

Health and wellness coaching is governed by a national board (nbhwc.org) who, in conjunction with the National Board of Medical Examiners, created a national exam for board certification. Coaches who are nationally board-certified have passed a rigorous testing process. Although they are not required to choose a specialty or concentration, many coaches have made brain health their area of focus. The National Board for Health and Wellness Coaching has a directory, and healthcare providers may be able to provide a referral. If you do an internet search using descriptive words and a city, be sure to speak with coaches who are board-certified and can explain how they will work with you (how often you will meet, their fees, and their approach). Ask about their experience and whether they have worked with clients who have issues similar to your own.

Other Specialized Websites
For a specific health condition, you may be able to narrow down your search. For example, if you are suffering from mold exposure or toxicity, survivingmold.com may provide valuable information as well as how to locate a qualified doctor for treatment.

Do an Internet Search for Integrative Doctors in Your Area
Many search engines are designed to offer listings by location, and those in your area are likely to come up at the top of the list. Follow the suggestions mentioned previously.

Contact Apollo Health (apollohealthco.com)
For those who want comprehensive testing, assignment of a trained practitioner, access to a health coach, and additional resources and groups to help support them on their path to cognitive health, Dr. Dale Bredesen's Apollo Health is an option. It provides one-stop shopping for diagnosis and most types of treatment, although other specialty trained doctors may be necessary.

14

Additional Reading

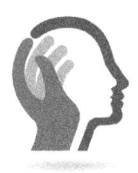

Aging Well

Outlive: The Science and Art of Longevity by Bill Gifford and Peter Attia, MD

The Longevity Paradox: How to Die Young at a Ripe Old Age by Steven R. Gundry, MD

The New Rules of Aging Well: A Simple Program for Immune Resilience, Strength, and Vitality by Frank Lipman, MD

Autoimmune Disease

The Plant Paradox by Steven R. Gundry, MD

The Wahls Protocol (2020) by Terry Wahls, MD

Brain Health

The End of Alzheimer's by Dale Bredesen, MD

The End of Alzheimer's Program by Dale Bredesen, MD, with Julie Gregory and Aida Lasheen Bredesen, MD

The Brain that Changes Itself by Norman Doidge, MD

Keep Sharp: How to Build a Better Brain at Any Age by Sanjay Gupta, MD

The UltraMind Solution by Mark Hyman, MD

The XX Brain by Lisa Mosconi, PhD

Brain Maker by David Perlmutter, MD

The Alzheimer's Solution by Ayesha Sherzai, MD, and Dean Sherzai, MD

Cardiovascular Health

What Your Doctor May Not Tell You About Heart Disease by Mark Houston, MD

Personalized and Precision Integrative Cardiovascular Medicine by Mark Houston, MD

Hormones

Stop the Thyroid Madness by Janie Bowthorpe, MEd

The Menopause Brain by Lisa Mosconi, PhD

Hashimoto's Thyroiditis: Lifesty;e Interventions for Finding and Treating the Root Cause by Izabella Wentz, PharmD

Nutrition

Ketotarian by Will Cole, DC

Wheat Belly by William Davis, MD

Super Immunity by Joel Fuhrman, MD

The Brain Body Diet by Sara Gottfried, MD

How Not to Die by Michael Greger, MD

Food: What the Heck Should I Eat? by Mark Hyman, MD

The Longevity Diet by Valter Longo, PhD

The Healthy Brain Solution for Women Over Forty by Nancy Lonsdorf, MD

Fat for Fuel by Joseph Mercola, DO

KetoFast by Joseph Mercola, DO

Grain Brain by David Perlmutter, MD

31-Day Food Revolution by Ocean Robbins

Personal Stories of Regaining Cognition

Alzheimer's Unmasked by Paul Barton

The First Survivors of Alzheimer's by Dale Bredesen, MD

Defeating Dementia by Frank McNear

Beating Alzheimer's: A Step Towards Unlocking the Mysteries of Brain Diseases by Tom Warren

Sleep and Breathing

GASP by Michael Gelb, DDS, and Howard Hindin, DDS

The Sleep Revolution by Arianna Huffington

Breath by James Nestor

Why We Sleep by Matthew Walker, PhD

Stress

Stress Less, Accomplish More by Emily Fletcher

Resilient by Rick Hanson, PhD

Thrive by Arianna Huffington

Wherever You Go There You Are by Jon Kabat-Zinn, PhD

Brain Wash by David Perlmutter, MD

Toxins

Non-Toxic: Guide to Living Healthy in a Chemical World by Aly Cohen, MD, and Frederick vom Saal, PhD

Toxic Beauty by Samuel S. Epstein, MD

Wired for Healing by Annie Hopper

How Can I Get Better? An Action Plan for Treating Resistant Lyme and Chronic Disease by Richard Horowitz, MD

The Lyme Solution by Darin Ingels, ND

Toxic: Heal Your Body by Neil Nathan, MD

The Toxin Solution by Joseph Pizzorno, ND

Toxic Legacy by Stephanie Seneff, PhD

Surviving Mold by Ritchie Shoemaker, MD

Trauma

Textbook of Traumatic Brain Injury, 3rd Edition, edited by Jonathan M. Silver, MD, Thomas W. Mcallister, MD, and David B. Arciniegas, MD

The Body Keeps the Score by Bessel van der Kolk, MD

Acknowledgments

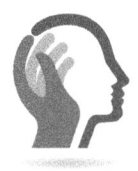

THIS BOOK TOOK SHAPE and changed as our knowledge of the brain's capabilities became better known over the past 12 years. The initial chapters were drafted by members of the Sharp Again Medical Advisory Board who have decades of experience in their respective fields and possess a strong desire to understand the underlying causes of disease. We are indebted to Richard Carlton, MD, Howard Hindin, DDS, Robert Kachko, ND, LAc, Gary Klingsberg, DO, Cornelia Lenherr, MD, Susanne Saltzman, MD, David Lerner, DDS, Michael Gelb, DDS, and Allan Warshowsky, MD, for their initial contributions and subsequent review of the materials.

Over several years, the advisory board, members of the Sharp Again board, and research and editorial volunteers worked on the project. As Minding Your Memory found its current form and chapters were added, additional members of the advisory board provided their input and review. Shanhong Lu, MD, Penelope McDonnell, ND, and Ilene Naomi Rusk, PhD, contributed their time, knowledge, and experience to help ensure that this book presents the most relevant and up-to-date information.

Barbara Goldenberg deserves special recognition for her editing, research, and the long hours spent working side by side with the editors to ready the book for publication.

Additional Sharp Again board members and volunteers who donated their time include Jacqui Bishop, Jennifer Hahn, Henry Sobo, MD, and Nancy Weiser, MBA, NBC-HWC.

We appreciate Karel Karpe and Joan Benz for their time and efforts in supporting Sharp Again and this project.

A special thank you goes to Patricia Tamowski and Alan Scott Douglas for their efforts in researching and filming individuals, their family members, doctors, and researchers who were on the front lines of understanding that memory loss has actual causes and who showed that memory could be restored. Without their time and efforts, Sharp Again would not exist today.

We could not have been more fortunate in working with Peggy Nehmen, Andrew Doty, and Allison Janicki on the development, copyediting, and design of the book. Their expertise in leading us through the publishing process has brought Minding Your Memory to fruition.

Glossary

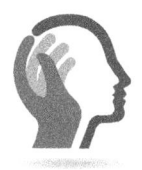

A

Acetyl-L-Carnitine: A nutrient that supports brain health and energy metabolism and is often used as a supplement for traumatic brain injury patients to improve cognitive function.

Adrenal Gland: Triangular-shaped glands that sit atop the kidneys and secrete a wide variety of hormones.

Adverse Childhood Experiences (ACEs): Early-life experiences such as abuse, neglect, or household dysfunction that have long-term effects on an individual's health, memory, and cognitive function later in life.

Allele: A variant of a gene.

Amalgam Fillings: Dental restorations that contain mercury, silver, and other metals. Mercury from these fillings can release vapor into the body, leading to potential toxicity.

Amygdala: A small, almond-shaped structure in the brain that processes emotion.

Amyloid Beta: A peptide that is a primary aspect of the plaques that build up in the brain.

Antibodies: Proteins produced by B-cells that are activated after being exposed to an antigen and which activate an immune response.

Antioxidant: Oxidation is a natural process that occurs when oxygen is metabolized and creates free radicals, which can cause damage to DNA and other cells. Antioxidants are substances that protect cells from the damage caused by free radicals. Foods such as berries, dark leafy greens, green tea, and whole grains are high in antioxidants.

ApoE4 Gene: A genetic variant associated with an increased risk of developing Alzheimer's disease and reduced ability to excrete heavy metals.

Autoimmune Disease: A condition where the body mounts an immune response to healthy tissue, cells, and organs, causing inflammation in the body.

B

Balance Training: Exercises like yoga, Tai Chi, and Qigong that help improve balance and prevent falls and injuries, which is especially important after a traumatic brain injury.

Beta Amyloid: A protein that develops from the breakdown of the amyloid precursor protein and can be found between neurons. When it clumps together, it can impair neuronal functioning.

Bioidentical Hormones: Artificial hormones that are chemically the same as hormones produced by the body. These are often used to treat symptoms of menopause and may be compounded in a pharmacy or produced in a factory.

Bisphenol A (BPA): A chemical used to make resins and plastics.

Blood Lead Levels (BLLs): A measurement used to assess lead concentration in the blood.

Brain Fog: A state of mental confusion or lack of clarity. Symptoms include difficulty focusing, impaired memory, and challenges in completing tasks.

Brain-Derived Neurotrophic Factor (BDNF): A protein found in the brain and spinal cord that helps nerve cells grow and thrive.

C

Chelation: A treatment method that involves using substances to bind with heavy metals in the body, allowing them to be excreted through urine or stool.

Chronic Traumatic Encephalopathy (CTE): A progressive, degenerative brain disease found in individuals with a history of repeated head injuries that is commonly seen in athletes who play contact sports.

Citicoline: A supplement that supports brain repair and cognitive function by increasing the production of phosphatidylcholine, a major component of brain cell membranes.

Complex Post-Traumatic Stress Disorder (C-PTSD): A form of PTSD resulting from prolonged and repeated trauma, leading to emotional and cognitive challenges.

CoQ10 (Ubiquinone): A nutrient important for cellular energy production and healing. It is beneficial for managing periodontal disease and is affected by statin medications.

Cortisol: A stress hormone released in response to trauma or chronic stress, which can lead to cognitive issues, adrenal fatigue, and memory impairment.

C-Reactive Protein: A protein made by the liver that increases when there is inflammation or tissue damage in the body.

Curcumin: The active compound in turmeric with powerful anti-inflammatory and antioxidant properties, shown to reduce joint pain and swelling by blocking inflammatory pathways.

Cytokines: Small signaling proteins released by cells that have a specific effect on the interactions and communications between cells. They play crucial roles in immune responses, inflammation, cell growth, and regulation.

D

Delirium: An acute change in mental status, including confusion and altered consciousness, often seen in older adults with UTIs or other infections.

Dementia: A progressive disease that involves loss of memory and other cognitive abilities with an inability to perform normal functions.

Detox Pathways: Ways that the body removes toxins: primarily through the liver, kidneys, sweat, urine, and stool.

Detoxification: The body's natural process of ridding itself of harmful substances, mainly through the liver, sweat, urine, and stool.

Dietary Approaches to Stop Hypertension (DASH) Diet: An eating plan that helps to lower blood pressure and promotes weight loss.

Dissociation: A mental process where an individual feels detached from their surroundings, themselves, or their emotions and is often a coping mechanism for trauma.

E

Emotional Trauma: A psychological injury resulting from overwhelming distress or helplessness, often leading to long-term emotional and physiological effects on the nervous system and brain.

Endodontic Disease: An infection that begins inside the tooth and can spread to surrounding tissues and beyond, potentially causing systemic infections.

Epigenetics: The study of how trauma and environmental factors can cause changes in gene expression, which may be passed down to future generations.

Etiology: The cause of a disease.

Eye Movement Desensitization and Reprocessing (EMDR): A therapy that helps process trauma by using guided eye movements combined with focused recollection of traumatic events.

F

Flashbacks: Sudden and intense reliving of past traumatic events, often accompanied by vivid images, emotions, and body sensations.

Functional Medicine: A patient-centered approach that treats the body as a whole and focuses on wellness and the root cause of disease.

G

Galvanic Reaction: An electrochemical reaction that occurs when different metals, such as mercury and gold, are present in the mouth, increasing the toxicity of the mercury.

Ganglia: Groups of nerve cells that carry signals between the peripheral and central nervous system.

H

Heavy Metal Poisoning: A condition caused by the accumulation of heavy metals, such as mercury and lead, which can lead to numerous health issues, including cognitive decline and chronic illnesses.

Heavy Metals (HM): A group of elements with a high density that can be toxic even at low levels. Common heavy metals include mercury, lead, arsenic, and cadmium.

High-Sensitivity C-Reactive Protein (hs-CRP): A blood test used to detect chronic inflammation in the body.

Hippocampus: A seahorse-shaped part of the brain that is responsible for forming, storing, and processing memory.

Holistic: A treatment approach that looks at the whole person, including physical, mental, and emotional factors.

Homocysteine: An amino acid measured in the blood that can indicate vitamin deficiencies or heart disease. Elevated levels are associated with inflammation and an increased risk of cognitive decline.

Homozygotes: Individuals who have two copies of a particular allele of the same gene.

Hydrogenated Fat (also known as Trans Fat): A type of fat where hydrogen is added to unsaturated fat to increase a product's shelf life.

Hyperarousal: A heightened state of anxiety and stress that occurs when trauma triggers the nervous system. It often leads to re-experiencing the trauma and difficulty processing emotion.

Hyperbaric Oxygen Therapy (HBOT): A treatment that involves breathing pure oxygen in a pressurized room or chamber, used to accelerate healing in brain injuries by promoting cellular energy production.

Hypothalamus: A gland located deep in the brain that acts as the body's control center, keeping it in homeostasis.

Hypoxia: A condition where the body's tissues do not have enough oxygen.

I

Immunoglobulin E (IgE) Test: A test that measures immediate allergic responses to foods, often causing acute symptoms like hives or anaphylaxis.

Immunoglobulin G (IgG) Test: A blood test that detects delayed immune responses to foods, which can cause chronic inflammation and more systemic symptoms.

Inflammation: The body's natural response to injury or infection, often resulting in pain, heat, redness, or swelling. Chronic inflammation can contribute to diseases such as Alzheimer's and vascular dementia.

Insulin Receptors: Proteins on neurons that help transport glucose into cells. When these receptors are reduced in effectiveness, the brain struggles to use glucose as fuel, leading to cognitive decline.

Insulin Resistance: A condition that occurs when cells are not able to efficiently use glucose for energy.

Integrative Medicine: Originally a practice that incorporated both Eastern (Asian) and Western (American and European) health philosophies, it is now more commonly thought of as combining practices and treatments from alternative medicine with conventional medicine.

Interleukin-6 (IL-6): A protein produced at the site of inflammation that helps to regulate the immune system.

Intermittent Fasting: A period of time, varying in duration, where a person does not eat, thereby allowing the body's systems to regulate. Examples are alternate day fasting and a daily fast of 12 to 16 hours.

Interoception: The awareness of internal body sensations, often used in somatic therapies to help individuals connect with and process trauma stored in the body.

K

Ketogenic Diet: A diet high in protein and healthy fats and low in carbohydrates that puts the body in ketosis so that it is burning fat instead of glucose for fuel.

Ketones: Molecules produced from the breakdown of fats that are used as an alternative fuel for the brain when glucose cannot be utilized effectively, especially in conditions like TBI and Alzheimer's disease.

L

Leaky Gut: A condition where the intestinal lining becomes permeable, allowing particles and toxins to enter the bloodstream, leading to inflammation.

Lipids: Fatty compounds in the cells that regulate the movement of what enters and leaves the cells and are responsible for storage, signaling, and cell structure.

Longitudinal Study: A research study that follows the same group of human subjects over time to look at changes in characteristics or other variables as they age.

M

Mediterranean Diet: A health-promoting diet found in Mediterranean countries that consists of fruits, vegetables, whole grains, lean animal protein and fish, limited dairy products, and healthy fats such as nuts and seeds, avocados, and extra virgin olive oil.

Medium-Chain Triglycerides (MCT) Oil: A type of fat that is quickly converted into ketones by the liver, providing an alternative energy source for the brain.

Mercury: A neurotoxic heavy metal that can accumulate in fatty tissues and mimic diseases like Alzheimer's.

Mercury Amalgam Removal: The process of removing mercury-containing dental fillings, which should be done with appropriate precautions to minimize mercury exposure.

Mercury Toxicity: A condition resulting from exposure to mercury, which can cause a variety of symptoms and increase the risk for neurological diseases like Alzheimer's.

Meta-Analysis: A statistical method used in research that combines data from different studies to draw a single conclusion about a given topic.

Methylation Cycle: A process that facilitates many vital functions in the body, such as hormone metabolism, neurotransmitter production, organ health, and detoxification.

Methylmercury: A highly toxic form of mercury that accumulates in fish, especially large predators, and poses significant health risks when ingested.

Microbiome/Microbiota: Microorganisms in the body that exist in a particular environment in a state of balance and symbiosis (i.e., the gut microbiome, the oral microbiome).

Microglia: Cells that are part of the brain's immune system that monitor and respond to pathogens and damage.

Micronized Progesterone: A bioidentical hormone typically used in hormone replacement therapy that can also help reduce brain inflammation following a concussion or traumatic brain injury.

Mild Cognitive Impairment (MCI): A stage in the progression of cognitive decline when a person's cognitive abilities are not functioning within a normal range for their age but do not yet interfere with most activities of daily life.

Mitochondria: Organelles found in cell membranes that produce energy for the cell.

Multi-Therapeutic Approach: Treating a medical condition with more than one intervention at a time to address a wider number of underlying causes.

N

Neurodegenerative: The progressive degeneration of nerve cells in the body.

Neurodegenerative Diseases: A group of disorders, including Alzheimer's, Parkinson's, and multiple sclerosis, that involve the progressive degeneration of nerve cells.

Neurofeedback (NF): A biofeedback technique that trains individuals to regulate abnormal brain activity patterns, which can improve executive function after a traumatic brain injury.

Neurofibrillary Tangles: Abnormal accumulations of a protein called tau that collect inside neurons.

Neurogenesis: The process by which new neurons are formed in the brain.

Neuroinflammation: An inflammatory response in the brain and spinal cord that may be caused by infection, traumatic brain injury, or exposure to environmental toxins.

Neuron: A cell in the nervous system that transmits and receives signals.

Neuroplasticity: The brain's ability to reorganize and form new neural connections in response to experiences throughout life, which is critical for healing from trauma.

Neurotoxins: Substances that are poisonous or destructive to nerve tissue.

Neurotransmitter: A chemical messenger that facilitates communication between nerve cells and other cells in the body.

O

Omega-3 Fatty Acids: Essential fats found in fish oil that reduce inflammation, improve blood flow to the brain, and support healing of central nervous system cells.

Oxidative Stress: An imbalance between free radicals and antioxidants in the body, leading to cell and tissue damage and contributing to inflammation.

P

Parasympathetic Nervous System: The part of the autonomic nervous system responsible for rest, relaxation, and recovery, often activated through practices like yoga and deep breathing.

Parts per Billion (ppb): A measurement used to describe the concentration of substances, especially toxins, in small amounts.

Pathogenesis: The process by which a disease progresses.

Per- and Polyfluoroalkyl Substances (PFAS): Synthetic chemicals used in many products and known as "forever chemicals" because they don't break down easily in the environment.

Phosphorylated Tau (p-tau): A brain protein that may undergo abnormal chemical changes that form into tangles inside neurons, thereby blocking the neuron's transport system and interfering with signaling between neurons.

Phthalates: Chemicals used in creating plastics that are shown to be endocrine disruptors and have an adverse effect on human health.

Plasticizers: Additives such as bisphenol A and phthalates that soften plastic, making it resilient and elastic.

Post-Traumatic Stress Disorder (PTSD): A mental health condition triggered by experiencing or witnessing a traumatic event. Symptoms include flashbacks, nightmares, hypervigilance, and dissociation.

Prebiotics: Nondigestible fibers that feed beneficial gut bacteria that are found in foods like garlic, onions, and bananas.

Prefrontal Cortex: A part of the brain located in the frontal lobe that controls executive functioning, decision making, planning, and working memory.

Probiotics: Live beneficial bacteria that help maintain gut health. They are found in fermented foods like yogurt, kimchi, and sauerkraut.

R

Rapid Eye Movement (REM) Sleep: A stage of sleep usually beginning 90 minutes after falling asleep and characterized by a high level of brain activity and dreaming. REM sleep is important for consolidation of memories.

Receptor: A protein that resides on the membrane of a cell. They detect and monitor changes occurring inside and outside the body. In the brain, receptors enable cells to communicate with each other.

S

Silver/Mercury Amalgam Fillings: Dental restorations that contain mercury, which can release mercury vapor into the body over time.

Sympathetic Nervous System: The part of the autonomic nervous system that responds to danger, stress, and exercise by increasing heart rate, blood pressure, breathing rate, and pupil size. It also causes blood vessels to constrict and decreases digestive juices.

Synapse: A connection between neurons in the brain, allowing them to communicate with each other.

T

Telomerase: An enzyme that adds DNA to telomeres (the ends of chromosomes) to help keep cells alive.

Thimerosal: A mercury-based preservative used in some vaccines, which has raised concerns about mercury exposure.

Toxic Body Burden: The point at which the body has absorbed more toxins than it can safely eliminate, leading to a buildup in tissues and organs.

Toxicity: The degree to which a substance can cause harm to the body, often through overexposure or accumulation.

U

Urinary Tract Infections (UTIs): Infections that can cause systemic inflammation and cognitive issues, especially in older adults.

Endnotes

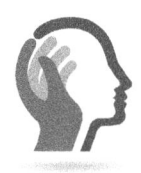

1. GBD 2019 Dementia Forecasting Collaborators. Estimation of the global prevalence of dementia in 2019 and forecasted prevalence in 2050: an analysis for the Global Burden of Disease Study 2019. *Lancet Public Health*. 2022 Feb; 7(2): e105–e125. doi: 10.1016/S2468-2667(21)00249-8.

2. Zhong G, Wang Y, Zhang Y, Guo JJ, Zhao Y. Smoking is associated with an increased risk of dementia: a meta-analysis of prospective cohort studies with investigation of potential effect modifiers. *PLoS One*. 2015 Mar 12; 10(3): e0118333. doi: 10.1371/journal.pone.0118333.

3. Tyas SL, White LR, Petrovitch H, et al. Mid-life smoking and late-life dementia: the Honolulu-Asia Aging Study. *Neurobiol Aging*. 2003 Jul–Aug; 24(4): 589–596. doi: 10.1016/s0197-4580(02)00156-2.

4. Tobacco & Dementia. World Health Organization. Published June 2014. Accessed March 25, 2025. https://iris.who.int/bitstream/handle/10665/128041/WHO_NMH_PND_CIC_TKS_14.1_eng.pdf.

5. Topiwala A, Valkanova V, Allan CL, et al. Moderate alcohol consumption as risk factor for adverse brain outcomes and cognitive decline: longitudinal cohort study. *BMJ*. 2017 Jun 6; 357: j2353. doi: 10.1136/bmj.j2353.

6. Livingston G, Huntley J, Sommerlad A, et al. Dementia prevention, intervention, and care: 2020 report of the Lancet Commission. *Lancet Public Health*. 2020 Aug 8; 396(10248): 413–446. doi: 10.1016/S0140-6736(20)30367-6.

7. Bredesen D, Sharlin K, Jenkins D, et al. Reversal of Cognitive Decline: 100 Patients. *J Alzheimers Dis Parkinsonism*. 2018; 8 (5). doi: 10.4172/2161-0460.1000450.

8. Rosenberg A, Mangialasche F, Ngandu T, Solomon A, Kivipelto M. Multidomain Interventions to Prevent Cognitive Impairment, Alzheimer's Disease, and Dementia: From FINGER to World-Wide FINGERS. *J Prev Alzheimers Dis*. 2020; 7(1): 29–36. doi: 10.14283/jpad.2019.41.

9. Toups K, Hathaway A, Gordon D, et al. Precision Medicine Approach to Alzheimer's Disease: Successful Pilot Project. *J Alzheimers Dis*. 2022; 88(4): 1411–1421. doi: 10.3233/JAD-215707.

10. Road Map to a Sharper Mind. Sharp Again. Accessed March 25, 2025. https://sharpagain.org/get-informed/get-started-now.

11. Kivipelto M, Solomon A, Ahtiluoto S, et al. The Finnish Geriatric Intervention Study to Prevent Cognitive Impairment and Disability (FINGER): study design and progress. *Alzheimers Dement*. 2013 Nov; 9(6): 657–665. doi: 10.1016/j.jalz.2012.09.012.

12. Ngandu T, Lehtisalo J, Solomon A, et al. A 2 year multidomain intervention of diet, exercise, cognitive training, and vascular risk monitoring versus control to prevent cognitive decline in at-risk elderly people (FINGER): a randomised controlled trial. *Lancet Public Health*. 2015 Jun 6; 385(9984): 2255–2263. doi: 10.1016/S0140-6736(15)60461-5.

13. Karp A, Paillard-Borg S, Silverstein M, Wang H. Mental, physical and social components in leisure activities equally contribute to decrease dementia risk. *Dement Geriatr Cogn Disord*. 2006 Feb. doi: 10.1159/000089919.

14. Coyle JT. Use it or lose it — do effortful mental activities protect against dementia? *N Engl J Med*. 2003 Jun 19; 348(25): 2489–2490. doi: 10.1056/NEJMp030051.

15. Bassuk SS, Manson JE. Epidemiological evidence for the role of physical activity in reducing risk of type 2 diabetes and cardiovascular disease. *J Appl Physiol* (1985). 2005 Sep; 99(3): 1193–1204. doi: 10.1152/japplphysiol.00160.2005.

16. Börjesson M, Onerup A, Lundqvist S, Dahlöf B. Physical activity and exercise lower blood pressure in individuals with hypertension: narrative review of 27 RCTs. *Br J Sports Med*. 2016 Mar; 50(6): 356–361. doi: 10.1136/bjsports-2015-095786.

17. Seeman TE. Social ties and health: the benefits of social integration. *Ann Epidemiol*. 1996; 6: 442–451. doi: 10.1016/s1047-2797(96)00095-6.

18. Rehfeld K, Müller P, Aye N, et al. Dancing or Fitness Sport? The Effects of Two Training Programs on Hippocampal Plasticity and Balance Abilities in Healthy Seniors. *Front Hum Neurosci*. 2017 Jun 15; 11: 305. doi: 10.3389/fnhum.2017.00305.

19. Nagata K, Tsunoda K, Fujii Y, Jindo T, Okura T. Impact of exercising alone and exercising with others on the risk of cognitive impairment among older Japanese adults. *Arch Gerontol Geriatr*. 2023; 107: 104908. doi: 10.1016/j.archger.2022.104908.

20. Rieker JA, Reales JM, Muiños M, Ballesteros S. The Effects of Combined Cognitive-Physical Interventions on Cognitive Functioning in Healthy Older Adults: A Systematic Review and Multilevel Meta-Analysis. *Front Hum Neurosci*. 2022 Mar 24; 16: 838968. doi: 10.3389/fnhum.2022.838968.

21. Castaño LAA, Castillo de Lima V, Barbieri JF, et al. Resistance training combined with cognitive training increases brain derived Neurotrophic factor and improves cognitive function in healthy older adults. *Front Psychol*. 2022; 13: 870561. doi: 10.3389/fpsyg.2022.870561.

22. Schelke MW, Attia P, Palenchar DJ, et al. Mechanisms of Risk Reduction in the Clinical Practice of Alzheimer's Disease Prevention. *Front Aging Neurosci*. 2018 Apr 10; 10: 96. doi: 10.3389/fnagi.2018.00096.

23. Isaacson RS, Hristov H, Saif N, et al. Individualized clinical management of patients at risk for Alzheimer's dementia. *Alzheimers Dement*. 2019; 15(12): 1588–1602. doi: 10.1016/j.jalz.2019.08.198.

24. Morris MC, Tangney CC, Wang Y, Barnes LL, Bennett D, Aggarwal NT. MIND Diet Score More Predictive than DASH or Mediterranean Diet Scores. *Alzheimers Dement*. 2014 Jul; 10(4): 164. doi: 10.1016/j.jalz.2014.04.164.

25. Morris MC, Tangney, CC, Wang Y, Sacks FM, Bennett DA, Aggarwal NT. MIND diet associated with reduced incidence of Alzheimer's disease. *Alzheimers Dement*. 2015 Sep; 11(9): 1007–1014. doi: 10.1016/j.jalz.2014.11.009.

26. van den Brink AC, Brouwer-Brolsma EM, Berendsen AAM, van de Rest O. The Mediterranean, Dietary Approaches to Stop Hypertension (DASH), and Mediterranean-DASH Intervention for Neurodegenerative Delay (MIND) Diets Are Associated with Less Cognitive Decline and a Lower Risk of Alzheimer's Disease — A Review. *Adv Nutr*. 2019; 10(6): 1040–1065. doi: 10.1093/advances/nmz054.

27. Tangney CC, Li H, Wang Y, et al. Relation of DASH- and Mediterranean-like dietary patterns to cognitive decline in older persons. *Neurology*. 2014 Oct 14; 83(16): 1410–1416. doi: 10.1212/WNL.0000000000000884.

28. Morris MC, Tangney CC, Wang Y, Sacks FM, Bennett DA, Aggarwal NT. MIND diet associated with reduced incidence of Alzheimer's disease. *Alzheimers Dement*. 2015 Sep; 11(9): 1007–1014. doi: 10.1016/j.jalz.2014.11.009.

29. Isaacson RS, Hristov H, Saif N, et al. Individualized clinical management of patients at risk for Alzheimer's dementia. *Alzheimers Dement*. 2019; 15(12): 1588–1602. doi: 10.1016/j.jalz.2019.08.198.

30. Devore EE, Kang JH, Breteler MM, Grodstein F. Dietary intakes of berries and flavonoids in relation to cognitive decline. *Ann Neurol*. 2012; 72(1): 135–143. doi: 10.1002/ana.23594.

31. Cao C, Cirrito J, Lin X, et al. Caffeine suppresses amyloid-β levels in plasma and brain of Alzheimer's disease transgenic mice. *J Alzheimers Dis*. 2009; 17(3): 681–697. doi: 10.3233/JAD-2009-1071.

32. Cao C, Loewenstein D, Lin X, et al. High blood caffeine levels in MCI linked to lack of progression to dementia. *J Alzheimers Dis*. 2012; 30(3): 559–572. doi: 10.3233/JAD-2009-1071.

33. Croteau E, Castellano C-A, Richard MA, et al. Ketogenic Medium Chain Triglycerides Increase Brain Energy Metabolism in Alzheimer's Disease. *J Alzheimers Dis*. 2018; 64(2): 551–561. doi: 10.3233/JAD-180202.

34. Isaacson RS, Ochner CN. *The Alzheimer's Prevention & Treatment Diet*. Square One Publishing; 2016: 174.

35. Bredesen DE. Reversal of cognitive decline: A novel therapeutic program. *Aging*. 2014 Sep. doi: 10.18632/aging.100690.

36. Qiu C, Winblad B, Marengoni A, et al. Heart Failure and Risk of Dementia and Alzheimer Disease: A Population-Based Cohort Study. *Arch Intern Med*. 2006; 166(9): 1003–1008. doi: 10.1001/archinte.166.9.1003.

37. Panickar KS. Beneficial effects of herbs, spices and medicinal plants on the metabolic syndrome, brain and cognitive function. *Cent Nerv Syst Agents Med Chem*. 2013 Mar; 13(1): 13–29. doi: 10.2174/1871524911313010004.

38 Liu Q, Meng X, Li Y, et al. Antibacterial and antifungal activities of spices. *Int J Mol Sci*. 2017 Jun; 18(6): 1283. doi: 10.3390/ijms18061283.

39 Aggarwal BB, Harikumar KB. Potential therapeutic effects of curcumin, the anti-inflammatory agent, against neurodegenerative, cardiovascular, pulmonary, metabolic, autoimmune and neoplastic diseases. *Int J Biochem Cell Biol*. 2009 Jan; 41(1): 40–59. doi: 10.1016/j.biocel.2008.06.010.

40 Ayati Z, Yang G, Ayati MH, Emani SA, Chang D. Saffron for mild cognitive impairment and dementia: a systematic review and meta-analysis of randomised clinical trials. *BMC Complement Med Ther*. 2020; 20(333). doi: 10.1186/s12906-020-03102-3.

41 Choudhary D, Bhattacharyya S, Bose S. Efficacy and Safety of Ashwagandha (*Withania somnifera* (L.) *Dunal*) Root Extract in Improving Memory and Cognitive Functions. *J Diet Suppl*. 2017 Nov 2; 14(6): 599–612. doi: 10.1080/19390211.2017.1284970.

42 Bacopa AIDS Memory, Cognition, Multitasking. *Journal of Plant Medicines*. Accessed March 25, 2025. https://plantmedicines.org/bacopa-memory-cognition-multitasking.

43 Roussel R, Fezeu L, Bouby N, et al. Low water intake and risk for new-onset hyperglycemia. *Diabetes Care*. 2011; 34(12): 2551–2554. doi: 10.2337/dc11-0652.

44 Omar SH. Mediterranean and MIND Diets Containing Olive Biophenols Reduces the Prevalence of Alzheimer's Disease. *Int J Mol Sci*. 2019 Jun 7; 20(11): 2797. doi: 10.3390/ijms20112797.

45 van den Brink AC, Brouwer-Brolsma EM, Berendsen AAM, van de Rest O. The Mediterranean, Dietary Approaches to Stop Hypertension (DASH), and Mediterranean-DASH Intervention for Neurodegenerative Delay (MIND) Diets Are Associated with Less Cognitive Decline and a Lower Risk of Alzheimer's Disease — A Review. *Adv Nutr*. 2019; 10(6): 1040–1065. doi: 10.1093/advances/nmz054.

46 What Are Prebiotics and What Do They Do? Cleveland Clinic. Published March 14, 2022. Accessed March 25, 2025. https://health.clevelandclinic.org/what-are-prebiotics.

47 Kim CS, Cha L, Sim M, Jung S, Chun WY, Baik HW, Shin DM. Probiotic Supplementation Improves Cognitive Function and Mood with Changes in Gut Microbiota in Community-Dwelling Older Adults: A Randomized, Double-Blind, Placebo-Controlled, Multicenter Trial. *J Gerontol A Biol Sci Med Sci*. 2021 Jan 1; 76(1): 32–40. doi: 10.1093/gerona/glaa090.

48 Akbari E, Asemi Z, Daneshvar KR, et al. Effect of Probiotic Supplementation on Cognitive Function and Metabolic Status in Alzheimer's Disease: A Randomized, Double-Blind and Controlled Trial. *Front Aging Neurosci*. 2016; 8. doi: 10.3389/fnagi.2016.00256 .

49 Liu N, Yang D, Sun J, Li Y. Probiotic supplements are effective in people with cognitive impairment: a meta-analysis of randomized controlled trials. *Nutr Rev*. 2023 Aug 10; 81(9): 1091–1104. doi: 10.1093/nutrit/nuac113.

50 Morris MC, Tangney CC, Wang Y, Sacks FM, Bennett DA, Aggarwal NT. MIND diet associated with reduced incidence of Alzheimer's disease. *Alzheimers Dement*. 2015 Sep; 11(9): 1007–1014. doi: 10.1016/j.jalz.2014.11.009.

51 Isaacson RS, Hristov H, Saif N, et al. Individualized clinical management of patients at risk for Alzheimer's dementia. *Alzheimers Dement*. 2019; 15(12): 1588–1602. doi: 10.1016/j.jalz.2019.08.198.

52. Raji CA, Erickson KI, Lopez OL, et al. Regular Fish Consumption and Age-Related Brain Gray Matter Loss. *Am J Prev Med*. 2014. doi: 10.1016/j.amepre.2014.05.037.

53. Neafsey EJ, Collins MA. Moderate alcohol consumption and cognitive risk. *Neuropsychiatr Dis Treat*. 2011; 7: 465. doi: 10.2147/NDT.S23159.

54. Daviet R, Aydogan G, Jagannathan K, et al. Associations between alcohol consumption and gray and white matter volumes in the UK Biobank. *Nat Commun*. 2022; 13: 1175. doi: 10.1038/s41467-022-28735-5.

55. Daviet R, Aydogan G, Jagannathan K, et al. Associations between alcohol consumption and gray and white matter volumes in the UK Biobank. *Nat Commun*. 2022; 13: 1175. doi: 10.1038/s41467-022-28735-5.

56. Ridley NJ, Draper B, Withall A. Alcohol-related dementia: an update of the evidence. *Alzheimers Res Ther*. 2013 Jan 25; 5(1): 3. doi: 10.1186/alzrt157.

57. Isaacson RS, Ochner CN. *The Alzheimer's Prevention & Treatment Diet.* Square One Publishers; 2016.

58. Bredesen DE. Reversal of cognitive decline: A novel therapeutic program. *Aging*. 2014 Sep. doi: 10.18632/aging.100690.

59. Nigg JT, Lewis K, Edinger T, Falk M. Meta-analysis of attention-deficit/hyperactivity disorder or attention-deficit/hyperactivity disorder symptoms, restriction diet, and synthetic food color additives. *J Am Acad Child Adolesc Psychiatry*. 2012 Jan; 51(1): 86–97, e8. doi: 10.1016/j.jaac.2011.10.015.

60. Warner JO. Artificial food additives: hazardous to long-term health? *Arch Dis Child*. 2024 Oct 18; 109(11): 882–885. doi: 10.1136/archdischild-2023-326565.

61. Song Z, Song R, Liu Y, Wu Z, Zhang X. Effects of ultra-processed foods on the microbiota-gut-brain axis: The bread-and-butter issue. *Food Res Int*. 2023 May; 167: 112730. doi: 10.1016/j.foodres.2023.112730.

62. Desideri G, Kwik-Uribe C, Grassi D, et al. Benefits in cognitive function, blood pressure, and insulin resistance through cocoa flavanol consumption in elderly subjects with mild cognitive impairment: the Cocoa, Cognition, and Aging (CoCoA) study. *Hypertension*. 2012 Sep; 60(3): 794–801. doi: 10.1161/HYPERTENSIONAHA.

63. Francis ST, Head K, Morris PG, Macdonald IA. The effect of flavanol-rich cocoa on the fMRI response to a cognitive task in healthy young people. *J Cardiovasc Pharmacol*. 2006; 47(2): S215–S220. doi: 10.1097/00005344-200606001-00018.

64. Lamport DJ, Christodoulou E, Achilleos C. Beneficial Effects of Dark Chocolate for Episodic Memory in Healthy Young Adults: A Parallel-Groups Acute Intervention with a White Chocolate Control. *Nutrients*. 2020 Feb 14; 12(2): 483. doi: 10.3390/nu12020483.

65. Socci V, Tempesta D, Desideri G, De Gennaro L, Ferrara M. Enhancing human cognition with cocoa flavonoids. *Front Nutr*. 2017; 4: 19. doi: 10.3389/fnut.2017.00019.

66. Lead and Cadmium Could Be in Your Dark Chocolate. *Consumer Reports*. Published December 15, 2022. Accessed March 25, 2025. https://www.consumerreports.org/health/food-safety/lead-and-cadmium-in-dark-chocolate-a8480295550.

67 Parke DV, Parke AL. Chemical-induced inflammation and inflammatory diseases. *Int J Occup Med Environ Health*. 1996; 9(3): 211–217.

68 Isaacson RS, Hristov H, Saif N, et al. Individualized clinical management of patients at risk for Alzheimer's dementia. *Alzheimers Dement*. 2019; 15(12): 1588–1602. doi: 10.1016/j.jalz.2019.08.198.

69 Richardson JR, Roy A, Shalat SL, et al. Elevated serum pesticide levels and risk for Alzheimer's disease. *JAMA Neurology*. 2014. 71(3): 284–290. doi: 10.1001/jamaneurol.2013.6030.

70 Bhave VM, Oladele CR, Ament Z, et al. Associations Between Ultra-Processed Food Consumption and Adverse Brain Health Outcomes. *Neurology*. 2024 Jun 11; 102(11): e209432. doi: 10.1212/WNL.0000000000209432.

71 Gomes Gonçalves N, Vidal Ferreira N, Khandpur N, et al. Association Between Consumption of Ultraprocessed Foods and Cognitive Decline. *JAMA Neurology*. 2023; 80(2): 142–150. doi:10.1001/jamaneurol.2022.4397.

72 Weinstein G, Vered S, Ivancovsky-Wajcman D, et al. Consumption of Ultra-Processed Food and Cognitive Decline among Older Adults With Type-2 Diabetes. *J Gerontol A Biol Sci Med Sci*. 2023 Jan 26; 78(1): 134–142. doi: 10.1093/gerona/glac070.

73 Perlmutter D. *Grain Brain*. Little, Brown Spark; 2018.

74 How much sodium should I eat per day? Heart.org. Updated January 5, 2024. Accessed February 15, 2020. https://www.heart.org/en/healthy-living/healthy-eating/eat-smart/sodium/how-much-sodium-should-i-eat-per-day.

75 Rush TM, Kritz-Silverstein D, Laughlin GA, Fung TT, Barrett-Connor E, McEvoy LK. Association between Dietary Sodium Intake and Cognitive Function in Older Adults. *J Nutr Health Aging*. 2017; 21(3): 276–283. doi: 10.1007/s12603-016-0766-2.

76 Pal K, Mukadam N, Petersen I, Cooper C. Mild cognitive impairment and progression to dementia in people with diabetes, prediabetes and metabolic syndrome: a systematic review and meta-analysis. *Soc Psychiatry Psychiatr Epidemiol*. 2018; 53: 1149–1160. doi: 10.1007/s00127-018-1581-3.

77 Bredesen D. *The End of Alzheimer's*. Avery; 2017: 50.

78 Jagust W. Is amyloid-β harmful to the brain? Insights from human imaging studies. *Brain*. 2016 Jan; 139(Pt 1): 23–30. doi: 10.1093/brain/awv326.

79 Debras C, Chazelas E, Sellem L, et al. Artificial sweeteners and risk of cardiovascular diseases: results from the prospective NutriNet-Santé cohort. *BMJ*. 2022; 378: e071204. doi: 10.1136/bmj-2022-071204.

80 Debras C, Deschasaux-Tanguy M, Chazelas E, et al. Artificial Sweeteners and Risk of Type 2 Diabetes in the Prospective NutriNet-Santé Cohort. *Diabetes Care*. 2023 Sep 1; 46(9): 1681–1690. doi: 10.2337/dc23-0206.

81 Glycemic index (GI) indicates how quickly a food increases blood sugar on a scale of 1–100 (pure glucose is 100). Glycemic load (GL) helps to understand a food's overall effect on blood sugar and takes into account the total amount of carbohydrates in food.

82   Laitinen MH, Ngandu T, Rovio S, et al. Fat Intake at Midlife and Risk of Dementia and Alzheimer's Disease: A Population-Based Study. *Dement Geriatr Cogn Disord*. 2006; 22: 99–107. doi: 10.1159/000093478.

83   Bhavsar N, St-Onge MP. The diverse nature of saturated fats and the case of medium-chain triglycerides: how one recommendation may not fit all. *Curr Opin Clin Nutr Metab Care*. 2016 Mar; 19(2): 81–87. doi: 10.1097/MCO.0000000000000249.

84   Luchsinger JA, Tang MX, Shea S, Mayeux R. Caloric intake and the risk of Alzheimer disease. *Arch Neurol*. 2002; 59(8): 1258–1263.

85   Gustafson D, Rothenberg E, Blennow K, Steen B, Skoog I. An 18-year follow-up of overweight and risk of Alzheimer disease. *Arch Intern Med*. 2003; 163(13): 1524–1528. doi: 10.1001/archinte.163.13.1524.

86   Geda YE, Ragossnig M, Roberts LA, et al. Caloric intake, aging, and mild cognitive impairment: a population-based study. *J Alzheimers Dis*. 2013; 34(2): 501–507. doi: 10.3233/JAD-121270.

87   Witte AV, Fobker M, Gellner R, Knecht S, Floel A. Caloric restriction improves memory in elderly humans. *Proc Natl Acad Sci USA*. 2009 Jan 27; 106(4): 1255–1260. doi: 10.1073/pnas.0808587106.

88   Isaacson RS, Ochner CN. *The Alzheimer's Prevention & Treatment Diet*. Square One Publishers; 2016.

89   Bredesen DE. Reversal of cognitive decline: A novel therapeutic program. *Aging*. 2014 Sep; 6(9): 707–717. doi: 10.18632/aging.100690.

90   de Cabo R, Mattson MP. Effects of Intermittent Fasting on Health, Aging, and Disease. *N Engl J Med*. 2019 Dec 26; 381(26): 2541–2551. doi: 10.1056/NEJMra1905136.

91   Krikorian R, Shidler M, Dangelo K, Couch SC, Benoit SC, Clegg DJ. Dietary ketosis enhances memory in mild cognitive impairment. *Neurobiol Aging*. 2012; 33(2): 425.e19–425.e27. doi: 10.1016/j.neurobiolaging.2010.10.006.

92   Fishel MA, Watson GS, Montine TJ, et al. Hyperinsulinemia provokes synchronous increases in central inflammation and β-amyloid in normal adults. *Arch Neurol*. 2005; 62(10): 1539–1544. doi: 10.1001/archneur.62.10.noc 50112.

93   D'Andrea Meira I, Romão TT, Pires do Prado HJ, Krüger LT, Pires MEP, da Conceição PO. Ketogenic Diet and Epilepsy: What We Know So Far. *Front Neurosci*. 2019 Jan 29; 13: 5. doi: 10.3389/fnins.2019.00005.

94   Annweiler CC. Low serum vitamin D concentrations in Alzheimer's disease: a systematic review and meta-analysis. *J Alzheimers Dis*. 2013; 33: 659–674. doi: 10.3233/JAD-2012-121432.

95   Littlejohns TJ, Henley WE, Lang IA, et al. Vitamin D and the risk of dementia and Alzheimer disease. *Neurology*. 2014; 83(10): 920–928. doi: 10.1212/WNL.0000000000000755.

96   Jadhav N, Ajgaonkar S, Saha P, et al. Molecular Pathways and Roles for Vitamin K2-7 as a Health-Beneficial Nutraceutical: Challenges and Opportunities. *Front Pharmacol*. 2022 Jun 14; 13: 896920. doi: 10.3389/fphar.2022.896920.

97   Dysken MW, Sano M, Asthana S, et al. Effect of Vitamin E and Memantine on Functional Decline in Alzheimer Disease: The TEAM-AD VA Cooperative Randomized Trial. *JAMA*. 2014; 311(1): 33–44. doi: 10.1001/jama.2013.282834.

98   Otsuka R, Tange C, Nishita Y, et al. Serum docosahexaenoic and eicosapentaenoic acid and risk of cognitive decline over 10 years among elderly Japanese. *Eur J Clin Nutr*. 2014; 68(4): 503–509. doi: 10.1038/ejcn.2013.264.

99   Yurko-Mauro K, Alexander DD, Van Elswyk ME. Docosahexaenoic Acid and Adult Memory: A Systematic Review and Meta-Analysis. *PLoS One*. 2015; 10(3): e0120391. doi: 10.1371/journal.pone.0120391.

100 Yurko-Mauro K. Beneficial effects of docosahexaenoic acid on cognition in age-related cognitive decline. *Alzheimers Dement*. 2010–2011; 6: 456–464. doi: 10.1016/j.jalz.2010.01.013.

101 Isaacson RS, Hristov H, Saif N, et al. Individualized clinical management of patients at risk for Alzheimer's dementia. *Alzheimers Dement*. 2019; 15(12): 1588–1602. doi: 10.1016/j.jalz.2019.08.198.

102 Bredesen D. *The End of Alzheimer's Program*. Penguin Publishing; 2020: 200.

103 World Health Organization. *Risk Reduction of Cognitive Decline*. January 2019.

104 Regular exercise changes the brain to improve memory, thinking skills. *Harvard Health*. Published April 9, 2014. Accessed March 25, 2025. https://www.health.harvard.edu/blog/regular-exercise-changes-brain-improve-memory-thinking-skills-201404097110.

105 Bredesen D. *The End of Alzheimer's Program*. Penguin Publishing; 2020: 201.

106 *Physical Activity Guidelines for Americans*, 2nd ed. Department of Health & Human Services. Published 2018. Accessed March 25, 2025. https://health.gov/sites/default/files/2019-09/Physical_Activity_Guidelines_2nd_edition.pdf.

107 Bredesen D. *The End of Alzheimer's*. Avery; 2017: 191.

108 Ahlskog JE, Geda YE, Graff-Radford NR, Petersen RC. Physical exercise as a preventive or disease-modifying treatment of dementia and brain aging. *Mayo Clin Proc*. 2011 Sep; 86(9): 876–884. doi: 10.4065/mcp.2011.0252.

109 Yamasaki T. Benefits of Table Tennis for Brain Health Maintenance and Prevention of Dementia. *Encyclopedia*. 2022; 2: 1577–1589. doi: 10.3390/encyclopedia2030107.

110 Yoon M, Yang P, Jin M, et al. Association of Physical Activity Level With Risk of Dementia in a Nationwide Cohort in Korea. *JAMA Network Open*. 2021; 4(12): e2138526. doi: 10.1001/jamanetworkopen.2021.38526.

111 Andel R, Crowe M, Pedersen NL, Fratiglioni L, Johansson B, Gatz M. Physical exercise at midlife and risk of dementia three decades later: a population-based study of Swedish twins. *J Gerontol A Biol Sci Med Sci*. 2008 Jan; 63(1): 62–66. doi: 10.1093/gerona/63.1.62.

112 Yamasaki T. Preventive Strategies for Cognitive Decline and Dementia: Benefits of Aerobic Physical Activity, Especially Open-Skill Exercise. *Brain Sci*. 2023 Mar 21; 13(3): 521. doi: 10.3390/brainsci13030521.

113 Erickson KI, Voss MW, Prakash RS, et al. Exercise training increases size of hippocampus and improves memory. *Proc Natl Acad Sci USA*. 2011 Feb 15; 108(7): 3017–322. doi: 10.1073/pnas.1015950108.

114 Pereira AC, Huddleston DE, Brickman AM, et al. An *in vivo* correlate of exercise-induced neurogenesis in the adult dentate gyrus. *Proc Natl Acad Sci USA*. 2007; 104(13): 5638–5643. doi: 10.1073/pnas.0611721104.

115 Stern Y, MacKay-Brandt A, Lee S, et al. Effect of aerobic exercise on cognition in younger adults. *Neurology*. 2019 Feb; 92(9): e905–e916. doi: 10.1212/WNL.00000000000070.

116 Sofi F, Valecchi D, Bacci D, et al. Physical activity and risk of cognitive decline: a meta-analysis of prospective studies. *J Intern Med*. 2011 Jan; 269(1): 107–117. doi: 10.1111/j.1365-2796.2010.02281.x.

117 Ahlskog JE, Geda YE, Graff-Radford NR, Petersen RC. Physical exercise as a preventive or disease-modifying treatment of dementia and brain aging. *Mayo Clin Proc*. 2011 Sep; 86(9): 876–884. doi: 10.4065/mcp.2011.0252.

118 Gibbons TD, Cotter JD, Ainslie PN, et al. Fasting for 20 h does not affect exercise-induced increases in circulating BDNF in humans. *J Physiol*. 2023 Jun; 601(11): 2121–2137. doi: 10.1113/JP283582.

119 Ai J-Y, Chen F-T, Hsieh S-S, et al. The Effect of Acute High-Intensity Interval Training on Executive Function: A Systematic Review. *Int J Environ Res Public Health*. 2021; 18(7): 3593. doi: 10.3390/ijerph18073593.

120 Mekari S, Neyedli HF, Fraser S, et al. High-Intensity Interval Training Improves Cognitive Flexibility in Older Adults. *Brain Sci*. 2020; 10(11): 796. doi: 10.3390/brainsci10110796.

121 Liu-Ambrose T, Nagamatsu LS, Graf P, Beattie BL, Ashe MC, Handy TC. Resistance Training and Executive Functions: A 12-Month Randomized Controlled Trial. *Arch Intern Med*. 2010; 170(2): 170–178. doi: 10.1001/archinternmed.2009.494.

122 Broadhouse KM, Singh MF, Suo C, et al. Hippocampal plasticity underpins long-term cognitive gains from resistance exercise in MCI. *Neuroimage: Clin*. 2020; 25: 102182. doi: 10.1016/j.nicl.2020.102182.

123 Herold F, Törpel A, Schega L, Müller NG. Functional and/or structural brain changes in response to resistance exercises and resistance training lead to cognitive improvements – a systematic review. *Eur Rev Aging Phys Act*. 2019 Jul 10; 16: 10. doi: 10.1186/s11556-019-0217-2.

124 Zunner BEM, Wachsmuth NB, Eckstein ML, et al. Myokines and Resistance Training: A Narrative Review. *Int J Mol Sci*. 2022; 23(7): 3501. doi: 10.3390/ijms23073501.

125 Pandey A, Pandey A, Pandey AS, Bonsignore A, Auclair A, Poirier P. Impact of Yoga on Global Cardiovascular Risk as an Add-On to a Regular Exercise Regimen in Patients With Hypertension. *Can J Cardiol*. 2023 Jan; 39(1): 57–62. doi: 10.1016/j.cjca.2022.09.019.

126 Sanogo F, Xu K, Cortessis V, Weigensberg M, Watanabe RM. Mind- and body-based interventions improve glycemic control in patients with type 2 diabetes: a systematic review and data-analysis. *J Integ Complem Med*. 2023; 29(2). doi: 10.1089/jicm.2022.0586.

127 Tyagi A, Cohen M. Yoga and heart rate variability: A comprehensive review of the literature. *Int J Yoga*. 2016 Jul-Dec; 9(2): 97–113. doi: 10.4103/0973-6131.183712.

128 Bridges L, Sharma M. The Efficacy of Yoga as a Form of Treatment for Depression. *J Evid Based Complementary Altern Med*. 2017 Oct; 22(4): 1017–1028. doi: 10.1177/2156587217715927.

129 Gothe NP, Khan I, Hayes J, Erlenbach E, Damoiseaux JS. Yoga Effects on Brain Health: A Systematic Review of the Current Literature. *Brain Plast*. 2019 Dec 26; 5(1): 105–122. doi: 10.3233/BPL-190084.

130 Shivaji C, Meenakshi C, Kashinath M, Sanjib KP, Nagaratna R. Impact of Yoga on cognition and mental health among elderly: A systematic review. *Complement Ther Med*. 2020; 52: 10241. doi: 10.1016/j.ctim.2020.102421.

131 García-Garro PA, Hita-Contreras F, Martínez-Amat A, et al. Effectiveness of a Pilates Training Program on Cognitive and Functional Abilities in Postmenopausal Women. *Int J Environ Res Public Health*. 2020; 17(10): 3580. doi: 10.3390/ijerph17103580.

132 Mello NF, Costa DL, Vasconcellos SV, Lensen CMM, Corazza ST. The effect of the contemporary Pilates method on physical fitness, cognition and promotion of quality of life among the elderly. *Rev Bras Geriatr Gerontol*. 2018 Sep–Oct; 21(05). doi: 10.1590/1981-22562018021.180083.

133 Park M, Song R, Ju K, et al. Effects of Tai Chi and Qigong on cognitive and physical functions in older adults: systematic review, meta-analysis, and meta-regression of randomized clinical trials. *BMC Geriatr*. 2023 Jun 6; 23(1): 352. doi: 10.1186/s12877-023-04070-2.

134 Kim TH, Pascual-Leone J, Johnson J, Tamim H. The mental-attention Tai Chi effect with older adults. *BMC Psychol*. 2016 May 31; 4(1): 29. doi: 10.1186/s40359-016-0137-0.

135 Wang Y, Tian J, Yang Q. Tai Chi exercise improves working memory capacity and emotion regulation ability. *Front Psychol*. 2023 Feb 16; 14: 1047544. doi: 10.3389/fpsyg.2023.1047544.

136 Tsang WW, Kwok JC, Hui-Chan CW. Effects of aging and tai chi on a finger-pointing task with a choice paradigm. *Evid Based Complement Alternat Med*. 2013; 653437. doi: 10.1155/2013/653437.

137 Chen Y, Qin J, Tao L, et al. Effects of Tai Chi Chuan on Cognitive Function in Adults 60 Years or Older With Type 2 Diabetes and Mild Cognitive Impairment in China: A Randomized Clinical Trial. *JAMA Network Open*. 2023; 6(4): e237004. doi:10.1001/jamanetworkopen.2023.7004.

138 Jasim N, Balakirishnan D, Zhang H, Steiner-Lim GZ, Karamacoska D, Yang GY. Effects and mechanisms of Tai Chi on mild cognitive impairment and early-stage dementia: a scoping review. *Syst Rev*. 2023 Oct 28; 12(1): 200. doi: 10.1186/s13643-023-02358-3.

139 Liu J, Shi H, Lee TM. Qigong exercise and cognitive function in brain imaging studies: a systematic review of randomized controlled trials in healthy and cognitively impaired populations. *Brain Behav Immun*. 2023; 3: 100016. doi: 10.1016/j.bbii.2023.100016.

140 Qi D, Wong NML, Shao R, et al. Qigong exercise enhances cognitive functions in the elderly via an interleukin-6-hippocampus pathway: A randomized active-controlled trial. *Brain Behav Immun*. 2021 Jul; 95: 381–390. doi: 10.1016/j.bbi.2021.04.011.

141 Isaacson RS, Hristov H, Saif N, et al. Individualized clinical management of patients at risk for Alzheimer's dementia. *Alzheimers Dement*. 2019; 15(12): 1588–1602. doi: 10.1016/j.jalz.2019.08.198.

142 Leanos S, Kurum E, Ditta A, Rebok G, Wu R. The impact of learning multiple new skills on cognitive development and functional independence in older adulthood. *Innov Aging*. 2018 Nov 16; 2(Suppl 1): 1004. doi: 10.1093/geroni/igy031.3708.

143 Clare L, Woods B. Cognitive rehabilitation and cognitive training for early-stage Alzheimer's disease and vascular dementia. *Cochrane Database Syst Rev.* 2003; (4): CD003260. doi: 10.1002/14651858. CD003260.

144 Ball K, Berch DB, Helmers KF, et al. Effects of cognitive training interventions with older adults: a randomized controlled trial. *JAMA.* 2002; 288: 2271–2281. doi: 10.1001/jama.288.18.2271.

145 Krell-Roesch J, Vemuri P, Pink A, et al. Association Between Mentally Stimulating Activities in Late Life and the Outcome of Incident Mild Cognitive Impairment, With an Analysis of the APOE ε4 Genotype. *JAMA Neurol.* 2017 Mar 1; 74(3): 332–338. doi: 10.1001/jamaneurol.2016.3822.

146 Kivipelto M, Solomon A, Ahtiluoto S, et al. The Finnish Geriatric Intervention Study to Prevent Cognitive Impairment and Disability (FINGER): study design and progress. *Alzheimers Dement.* 2013 Nov; 9(6): 657–665. doi: 10.1016/j.jalz.2012.09.012.

147 Tennstedt SL, Unverzagt FW. The ACTIVE study: study overview and major findings. *J Aging Health.* 2013 Dec; 25(8 Suppl): 3S–20S. doi: 10.1177/0898264313518133.

148 Cheng ST. Cognitive Reserve and the Prevention of Dementia: the Role of Physical and Cognitive Activities. *Curr Psychiatry Rep.* 2016 Sep; 18(9): 85. doi: 10.1007/s11920-016-0721-2.

149 Stern Y. Cognitive reserve in ageing and Alzheimer's disease. *Lancet Neurol.* 2012 Nov; 11(11): 1006–1012. doi: 10.1016/S1474-4422(12)70191-6.

150 Tucker AM, Stern Y. Cognitive reserve in aging. *Curr Alzheimer Res.* 2011 Jun; 8(4): 354–360. doi: 10.2174/156720511795745320.

151 Bredesen D. *The End of Alzheimer's Program.* Penguin Publishing; 2020: 244–245.

152 Harmat L, Takács J, Bódizs R. Music improves sleep quality in students. *J Adv Nurs.* 2008 May; 62(3): 327–335. doi: 10.1111/j.1365-2648.2008.04602.x.

153 Holt-Lunstad J, Smith TB, Layton JB. Social relationships and mortality risk: a meta-analytic review. *PLoS Med.* 2010 Jul 27; 7(7): e1000316. doi: 10.1371/journal.pmed.1000316.

154 Isolation in Older Americans Brings Health Risks. *AARP.* Published March 4, 2019. Accessed March 25, 2025. https://www.aarp.org/health/conditions-treatments/info-2017/isolation-loneliness-impacts-seniors-fd.html.

155 Huang AR, Roth DL, Cidav T, et al. Social isolation and 9-year dementia risk in community-dwelling Medicare beneficiaries in the United States. *J Am Geriatr Soc.* 2023 Mar; 71(3): 765–773. doi: 10.1111/jgs.18140.

156 Marioni RE, Proust-Lima C, Amieva H, et al. Social activity, cognitive decline and dementia risk: a 20-year prospective cohort study. *BMC Public Health.* 2015 Oct 24; 15: 1089. doi: 10.1186/s12889-015-2426-6.

157 Foubert-Samier A, Le Goff M, Helmer C, et al. Change in leisure and social activities and risk of dementia in elderly cohort. *J Nutr Health Aging.* 2014 Dec; 18(10): 876–882. doi: 10.1007/s12603-014-0475-7.

158 Foubert-Samier A, Le Goff M, Helmer C, et al. Change in leisure and social activities and risk of dementia in elderly cohort. *J Nutr Health Aging*. 2014 Dec; 18(10): 876–882. doi: 10.1007/s12603-014-0475-7.

159 Norton MC, Smith KR, Østbye T, et al. Greater risk of dementia when spouse has dementia? The Cache County study. *J Am Geriatr Soc*. 2010 May; 58(5): 895–900. doi: 10.1111/j.1532-5415.2010.02806.x.

160 Ren Y, Savadlou A, Park S, Siska P, Epp JR, Sargin D. The impact of loneliness and social isolation on the development of cognitive decline and Alzheimer's Disease. *Front Neuroendocrinol*. 2023 Apr; 69: 101061. doi: 10.1016/j.yfrne.2023.101061.

161 Bubu OM, Andrade AG, Umasabor-Bubu OQ, et al. Obstructive sleep apnea, cognition and Alzheimer's disease: A systematic review integrating three decades of multidisciplinary research. *Sleep Med Rev*. 2020 Apr; 50: 101250. doi: 10.1016/j.smrv.2019.101250.

162 Yaffe K, Laffan AM, Harrison SL, et al. Sleep-Disordered Breathing, Hypoxia, and Risk of Mild Cognitive Impairment and Dementia in Older Women. *JAMA*. 2011; 306(6): 613–619. doi: 10.1001/jama.2011.1115.

163 Gelb M, Hindin H. *GASP: Airway Health, The Hidden Path to Wellness*. CreateSpace; 2016.

164 Colten HR, Altevogt BM, Institute of Medicine (US) Committee on Sleep Medicine and Research, eds. *Sleep Disorders and Sleep Deprivation: An Unmet Public Health Problem*. Washington (DC): National Academies Press (US); 2006.

165 Jiao L, Duan Z, Sangi-Haghpeykar H, Hale L, White DL, El-Serag HB. Sleep duration and incidence of colorectal cancer in postmenopausal women. *Br J Cancer*. 2013 Jan 15; 108(1): 213–221. doi: 10.1038/bjc.2012.561.

166 Punjabi NM, Shahar E, Redline S, Gottlieb DJ, Givelber R, Resnick HE. Sleep Heart Health Study Investigators. Sleep-disordered breathing, glucose intolerance, and insulin resistance: the Sleep Heart Health Study. *Am J Epidemiol*. 2004 Sep 15; 160(6): 521–530. doi: 10.1093/aje/kwh261.

167 Ancoli-Israel S, Klauber MR, Butters N, Parker L, Kripke DF. Dementia in institutionalized elderly: relation to sleep apnea. *J Am Geriatr Soc*. 1991 Mar; 39(3): 258–263. doi: 10.1111/j.1532-5415.1991.tb01647.x.

168 Controlled ZZZs. *Cleveland Clinic*. Updated June 19, 2023. Accessed March 25, 2025. https://my.clevelandclinic.org/health/body/12148-sleep-basics.

169 Osorio RS, Pirraglia E, Agüera-Ortiz LF, et al. Greater risk of Alzheimer's disease in older adults with insomnia. *J Am Geriatr Soc*. 2011 Mar; 59(3): 559–562. doi: 10.1111/j.1532-5415.2010.03288.x.

170 Walker M. *Why We Sleep: Unlocking the Power of Sleep and Dreams*. Scribner; 2017: 114–117.

171 Hurtado-Alvarado G, Domínguez-Salazar E, Pavon L, Velázquez-Moctezuma J, Gómez-González B. Blood-Brain Barrier Disruption Induced by Chronic Sleep Loss: Low-Grade Inflammation May Be the Link. *J Immunol Res*. 2016; 4576012. doi: 10.1155/2016/4576012.

172 Sforza E, Roche F. Chronic intermittent hypoxia and obstructive sleep apnea: an experimental and clinical approach. *Hypoxia (Auckl)*. 2016 Apr 27; 4: 99–108. doi: 10.2147/HP.S103091.

173 Kheirandish-Gozal L, Gozal D. Obstructive Sleep Apnea and Inflammation: Proof of Concept Based on Two Illustrative Cytokines. *Int J Mol Sci*. 2019 Jan 22; 20(3): 459. doi: 10.3390/ijms20030459.

174 Taheri S, Lin L, Austin D, Young T, Mignot E. Short sleep duration is associated with reduced leptin, elevated ghrelin, and increased body mass index. *PLoS Med*. 2004 Dec; 1(3): e62. doi: 10.1371/journal.pmed.0010062.

175 Shokri-Kojori E, Wang GJ, Wiers CE, et al. β-Amyloid accumulation in the human brain after one night of sleep deprivation. *Proc Natl Acad Sci USA*. 2018 Apr 24; 115(17): 4483–4488. doi: 10.1073/pnas.1721694115.

176 Foundation for Airway Health. *Finding Connor Deegan*. Published Mar 13, 2015. Accessed March 25, 2025. https://www.youtube.com/watch?v=ZX5s4WNXK3M.

177 Brady MF, Burns B. *Airway Obstruction*. StatPearls. Updated August 7, 2023. Accessed March 25, 2025. https://www.ncbi.nlm.nih.gov/books/NBK470562/.

178 Canessa N, Castronovo V, Cappa SF, et al. Obstructive sleep apnea: brain structural changes and neurocognitive function before and after treatment. *Am J Respir Crit Care Med*. 2011 May 15; 183(10): 1419–1426. doi: 10.1164/rccm.201005-0693OC.

179 Gelb M, Hindin H. *GASP: Airway Health, The Hidden Path to Wellness*. CreateSpace; 2016.

180 Ancoli-Israel S, Palmer BW, Cooke JR, et al. Cognitive effects of treating obstructive sleep apnea in Alzheimer's disease: a randomized controlled study. *J Am Geriatr Soc*. 2008 Nov; 56(11): 2076–2081. doi: 10.1111/j.1532-5415.2008.01934.x.

181 Walker M. *Why We Sleep: Unlocking the Power of Sleep and Dreams*. Scribner; 2017: 101.

182 Walker M. *Why We Sleep: Unlocking the Power of Sleep and Dreams*. Scribner; 2017: 96.

183 Depner CM, Melanson EL, Eckel RH, et al. Ad libitum Weekend Recovery Sleep Fails to Prevent Metabolic Dysregulation during a Repeating Pattern of Insufficient Sleep and Weekend Recovery Sleep. *Curr Biol*. 2019 Mar 18; 29(6): 957–967. e4. doi: 10.1016/j.cub.2019.01.069.

184 Van Dongen HP, Maislin G, Mullington JM, Dinges DF. The cumulative cost of additional wakefulness: dose-response effects on neurobehavioral functions and sleep physiology from chronic sleep restriction and total sleep deprivation. *Sleep*. 2003 Mar 15; 26(2): 117–126. doi: 10.1093/sleep/26.2.117.

185 Walker M. *Why We Sleep: Unlocking the Power of Sleep and Dreams*. Scribner; 2017: 97.

186 For a complete list of the benefits of breastfeeding, see "101 Reasons to Breastfeed" at http://www.notmilk.com/11.html.

187 Redline S, Cook K, Chervin RD, et al. Adenotonsillectomy for snoring and mild sleep apnea in children: A randomized clinical trial. *JAMA*. 2023 Dec 5; 330(21): 2084–2095. doi: 10.1001/jama.2023.22114.

188 Huang YS, Guilleminault C. Pediatric obstructive sleep apnea and the critical role of oral-facial growth: evidences. *Front Neurol*. 2013 Jan 22; 3: 184. doi: 10.3389/fneur.2012.00184.

189   Kim DK, Rhee CS, Han DH, Won TB, Kim DY, Kim JW. Treatment of allergic rhinitis is associated with improved attention performance in children: the Allergic Rhinitis Cohort Study for Kids (ARCO-Kids). *PLoS One*. 2014 Oct 17; 9(10): e109145. doi: 10.1371/journal.pone.0109145.

190   Tosca MA, Licari A, Olcese R, et al. Allergen immunotherapy in children and adolescents with respiratory diseases. *Acta Biomed*. 2020 Sep 15; 91(11-S): e2020006. doi: 10.23750/abm.v91i11-S.10309.

191   Liu Y, Zhou JR, Xie SQ, Yang X, Chen JL. The Effects of Orofacial Myofunctional Therapy on Children with OSAHS's Craniomaxillofacial Growth: A Systematic Review. *Children (Basel)*. 2023 Mar 31; 10(4): 670. doi: 10.3390/children10040670.

192   Jezioro JR, Gutman SA, Lovinsky-Desir S, Rauh V, Perera FP, Miller RL. A Comparison of Activity Participation between Children with and without Asthma. *Open J Occup Ther*. 2021 Summer; 9(3): 12. doi: 10.15453/2168-6408.

193   Peter Attia, host. Matthew Walker, guest. *#58 – AMA with sleep expert, Matthew Walker, Ph.D.: Strategies for sleeping more, sleeping better, and avoiding things that are disrupting sleep*. 17 June 2019. https://peterattiamd.com/matthewwalkerama/.

194   Peter Attia, host. Matthew Walker, guest. *#58 – AMA with sleep expert, Matthew Walker, Ph.D.: Strategies for sleeping more, sleeping better, and avoiding things that are disrupting sleep*. 17 June 2019. https://peterattiamd.com/matthewwalkerama/.

195   Peter Attia, host. Matthew Walker, guest. *#58 – AMA with sleep expert, Matthew Walker, Ph.D.: Strategies for sleeping more, sleeping better, and avoiding things that are disrupting sleep*. 17 June 2019. https://peterattiamd.com/matthewwalkerama/.

196   Alzyoud A, AlShorman O, Masadeh M, Alkahtani F, Abdelrahman R. Learning and Memory under Stress: A Review Study with Evaluation Techniques. *Sys Rev Pharm*. 2021; 12(1): 1602–1610.

197   Fonken LK, Frank MG, Gaudet AD, Maier SF. Stress and aging act through common mechanisms to elicit neuroinflammatory priming. *Brain Behav Immun*. 2018; 73: 133–148. doi: 10.1016/j.bbi.2018.07.012.

198   Johansson L, Guo X, Waern M, et al. Midlife psychological stress and risk of dementia: a 35-year longitudinal population study. *Brain*. 2010 Aug; 133(Pt 8): 2217–2224. doi: 10.1093/brain/awq116.

199   Alshak MN, Das JM. Neuroanatomy, Sympathetic Nervous System. *StatPearls*. 2024 Jan. https://www.ncbi.nlm.nih.gov/books/NBK542195.

200   Harrison NA, Cercignani M, Voon V, Critchley HD. Effects of inflammation on hippocampus and substantia nigra responses to novelty in healthy human participants. *Neuropsychopharmacology*. 2015; 40(4): 831–838. doi: 10.1038/npp.2014.222.

201   Wallensten J, Ljunggren G, Nager A, et al. Stress, depression, and risk of dementia — a cohort study in the total population between 18 and 65 years old in Region Stockholm. *Alzheimers Res Ther*. 2023 Oct 2; 15(1): 161. doi: 10.1186/s13195-023-01308-4.

202   Joshi YB, Chu J, Praticò D. Stress hormone leads to memory deficits and altered tau phosphorylation in a model of Alzheimer's disease. *J Alzheimers Dis*. 2012; 31(1): 167–176. doi: 10.3233/JAD-2012-120328.

203 Wang Y, Li M, Tang J, et al. Glucocorticoids facilitate astrocytic amyloid-β peptide deposition by increasing the expression of APP and BACE1 and decreasing the expression of amyloid-β-degrading proteases. *Endocrinology*. 2011; 152(7): 2704-2715. doi: 10.1210/en.2011-0145.

204 University of California Irvine: Institute for Memory Impairments and Neurological Disorders. Stress and Its Influence on Alzheimer's Disease. UCIMIND. Published April 5, 2011. Accessed April 24, 2025. http://mind.uci.edu/stress-and-its-influence-on-alzheimers-disease/#sthash.Aa5idp5D.dpuf.

205 Rajmohan R, Reddy PH. Amyloid-Beta and Phosphorylated Tau Accumulations Cause Abnormalities at Synapses of Alzheimer's Disease Neurons. *J Alzheimers Dis*. 2017; 57(4): 975-999. doi: 10.3233/JAD-160612.

206 Ouanes S, Popp J. High Cortisol and the Risk of Dementia and Alzheimer's Disease: A Review of the Literature. *Front Aging Neurosci*. 2019 Mar 1; 11: 43. doi: 10.3389/fnagi.2019.00043.

207 de Souza-Talarico JN, Marin MF, Sindi S, Lupien SJ. Effects of stress hormones on the brain and cognition: Evidence from normal to pathological aging. *Dement Neuropsychol*. 2011 Jan-Mar; 5(1): 8-16. doi: 10.1590/S1980-57642011DN05010003.

208 Khalsa DS. Stress, Meditation, and Alzheimer's Disease Prevention: Where the Evidence Stands. *J Alzheimers Dis*. 2015; 48(1): 1-12. doi: 10.3233/JAD-142766.

209 Lavretsky H, Newhouse PA. Stress, inflammation, and aging. *Am J Geriatr Psychiatry*. 2012 Sep; 20(9): 729-733. doi: 10.1097/JGP.0b013e31826573cf.

210 *Stressful Life Experiences Age the Brain by Four Years, African Americans Most at Risk*. AAIC. Published July 16, 2017. Accessed March 25, 2025. https://www.alz.org/aaic/releases_2017/AAIC17-Sun-briefing-racial-disparities.asp.

211 *Women and Alzheimer's*. Alzheimer's Association. Accessed March 25, 2025. https://www.alz.org/alzheimers-dementia/what-is-alzheimers/women-and-alzheimer-s.

212 Lambrou NH, Gleason CE, Obedin-Maliver J, et al. Subjective Cognitive Decline Associated with Discrimination in Medical Settings among Transgender and Nonbinary Older Adults. *Int J Environ Res Public Health*. 2022 Jul 27; 19(15): 9168. doi: 10.3390/ijerph19159168.

213 Fredriksen-Goldsen KI, Kim H-J, Bryan AE, Shiu C, Emlet CA. The cascading effects of marginalization and pathways of resilience in attaining good health among LGBT older adults. *Gerontologist*. 2017; 57: S72-S83. doi: 10.1093/geront/gnw170.

214 Gouin JP, Glaser R, Malarkey WB, Beversdorf D, Kiecolt-Glaser. Chronic Stress, Daily Stressors, and Circulating Inflammatory Markers. *J Health Psychology*. 2012; 31(2): 264-268. doi: 10.1037/a0025536.

215 Linz R, Singer T, Engert V. Interactions of momentary thought content and subjective stress predict cortisol fluctuations in a daily life experience sampling study. *Sci Rep*. 2018 Oct 18; 8(1): 15462. doi: 10.1038/s41598-018-33708-0.

216 Ackerman SJ, Hilsenroth, MJ. A review of therapist characteristics and techniques positively impacting the therapeutic alliance. *Clin Psychol Rev*. 2003 Feb; 23(1): 1-33. doi: 10.1016/s0272-7358(02)00146-0.

217 Peavy GM, Lange KL, Salmon DP, et al. The effects of prolonged stress and APOE genotype on memory and cortisol in older adults. *Biol Psychiatry*. 2007 Sep 1; 62(5): 472–478. doi: 10.1016/j.biopsych.2007.03.013.

218 Lupien S, McEwen B, Gunnar M, et al. Effects of stress throughout the lifespan on the brain, behavior and cognition. *Nat Rev Neurosci*. 2009; 10: 434–445. doi: 10.1038/nrn2639.

219 Lupien S, Lecours AR, Lussier I, Schwartz G , Nair NP, Meaney MJ. Basal cortisol levels and cognitive deficits in human aging. *J of Neurosci*. 1994 May 1; 14(5): 2893–2903. doi: 10.1523/JNEUROSCI.14-05-02893.1994.

220 Lupien S, de Leon M, de Santi S, et al. Cortisol levels during human aging predict hippocampal atrophy and memory deficits. *Nat Neurosci*. 1998; 1: 69–73. doi: 10.1038/271.

221 Epel ES, Crosswell AD, Mayer SE, et al. More than a feeling: A unified view of stress measurement for population science. Front Neuroendocrinol. 2018 Apr; 49: 146–169. doi: 10.1016/j.yfrne.2018.03.001.

222 Wang HX, Wahlberg M, Karp A, Winblad B, Fratiglioni L. Psychosocial stress at work is associated with increased dementia risk in late life. *Alzheimers Dement*. 2012; 8(2): 114–120. doi: 10.1016/j.jalz.2011.03.001.

223 Wilson RS, Begeny CT, Boyle PA, Schneider JA, Bennett DA. Vulnerability to stress, anxiety, and development of dementia in old age. *Am J Geriatr Psychiatry*. 2011 Apr; 19(4): 327–334. doi: 10.1097/JGP.0b013e31820119da.

224 Heim C, Newport DJ, Miller AH, Nemeroff CB. Long-term neuroendocrine effects of childhood maltreatment. *JAMA*. 2000 Nov 8; 284(18): 2321.

225 Johansson L, Guo X, Hällström T, et al. Common psychosocial stressors in middle-aged women related to longstanding distress and increased risk of Alzheimer's disease: a 38-year longitudinal population study. *BMJ Open*. 2013; 3: e003142. doi: 10.1136/bmjopen-2013-003142.

226 Khoury B, Lecomte T, Fortin G, et al. Mindfulness-based therapy: a comprehensive meta-analysis. *Clin Psychol Rev*. 2013 Aug; 33(6): 763–771. doi: 10.1016/j.cpr.2013.05.005.

227 Hoge EA, Bui E, Marques L, et al. Randomized controlled trial of mindfulness meditation for generalized anxiety disorder: effects on anxiety and stress reactivity. *J Clin Psychiatry*. 2013 Aug; 74(8): 786–792. doi: 10.4088/JCP.12m08083.

228 Newberg AB, Wintering N, Khalsa DS, Roggenkamp H, Waldman MR. Meditation effects on cognitive function and cerebral blood flow in subjects with memory loss: a preliminary study. *J Alzheimers Dis*. 2010; 20(2): 517–526. doi: 10.3233/JAD-2010-1391.

229 Innes KE, Selfe TK, Brown CJ, Rose KM, Thompson-Heisterman A. The effects of meditation on perceived stress and related indices of psychological status and sympathetic activation in persons with Alzheimer's disease and their caregivers: a pilot study. *Evid Based Complement Alternat Med*. 2012; 2012: 927509. doi: 10.1155/2012/927509.

230 Khalsa DS, Amen D, Hanks C, Money N, Newberg A. Cerebral blood flow changes during chanting meditation. *Nucl Med Commun*. 2009 Dec; 30(12): 956–961. doi: 10.1097/MNM.0b013e32832fa26c.

231 Khalsa DS, Khalsa TK. The Pink Brain Project: How Yoga Meditation May Prevent Alzheimer's in Women. *Alzheimer's Association International Conference*. 2018 Jul 24. https://alz-journals.onlinelibrary.wiley.com/doi/pdf/10.1016/j.jalz.2018.06.1992.

232 Innes KE, Selfe TK, Brown CJ, Rose KM, Thompson-Heisterman A. The effects of meditation on perceived stress and related indices of psychological status and sympathetic activation in persons with Alzheimer's disease and their caregivers: a pilot study. *Evid Based Complement Alternat Med*. 2012; 2012: 927509. doi: 10.1155/2012/927509.

233 Innes KE, Selfe TK, Brundage K, et al. Z. Effects of Meditation and Music-Listening on Blood Biomarkers of Cellular Aging and Alzheimer's Disease in Adults with Subjective Cognitive Decline: An Exploratory Randomized Clinical Trial. *J Alzheimers Dis*. 2018; 66(3): 947–970. doi: 10.3233/JAD-180164.

234 Khalsa DS. Stress, Meditation, and Alzheimer's Disease Prevention: Where the Evidence Stands. *J Alzheimers Dis*. 2015; 48(1): 1–12. doi: 10.3233/JAD-142766.

235 Lavretsky H, Epel ES, Siddarth P, et al. A pilot study of yogic meditation for family dementia caregivers with depressive symptoms: effects on mental health, cognition, and telomerase activity. *Int J Geriatr Psychiatry*. 2013 Jan; 28(1): 57–65. doi: 10.1002/gps.3790.

236 Khalsa DS, Amen D, Hanks C, Money N, Newberg A. Cerebral blood flow changes during chanting meditation. *Nucl Med Commun*. 2009 Dec; 30(12): 956–961. doi: 10.1097/MNM.0b013e32832fa26c.

237 Khalsa DS. Yoga and Medical Meditation as Alzheimer's Prevention Medicine. White Paper. Accessed May 21, 2025. https://www.alzheimersprevention.org/downloadables/White_Paper.pdf.

238 Practice the 12-Minute Yoga Meditation Exercise. Alzheimer's Research & Prevention Foundation. Published July 20, 2022. Accessed March 25, 2025. https://alzheimersprevention.org/research/kirtan-kriya-yoga-exercise.

239 Wieland DR, Wieland JR, Wang H, et al. Thyroid Disorders and Dementia Risk: A Nationwide Population-Based Case-Control Study. *Neurology*. 2022 Aug 16; 99(7): e679–e687. doi: 10.1212/WNL.0000000000200740.

240 Maki PM, Henderson VW. Hormone therapy, dementia, and cognition: the Women's Health Initiative 10 years on. *Climacteric*. 2012 Jun; 15(3): 256–262. doi: 10.3109/13697137.2012.660613.

241 Bianchi VE. Impact of Testosterone on Alzheimer's Disease. *World J Mens Health*. 2022 Apr; 40(2): 243–256. doi: 10.5534/wjmh.210175.

242 Carroll JC, Rosario ER, Chang L, et al. Progesterone and estrogen regulate Alzheimer-like neuropathology in female 3xTg-AD mice. *J Neurosci*. 2007 Nov 28; 27(48): 13357–13365. doi: 10.1523/JNEUROSCI.2718-07.2007.

243 Ferguson EL, Zimmerman SC, Jiang C, et al. Low- and High-Density Lipoprotein Cholesterol and Dementia Risk Over 17 Years of Follow-up Among Members of a Large Health Care Plan. *Neurology*. 2023 Nov 21; 101(21): e2172–e2184. doi: 10.1212/WNL.0000000000207876.

244 Yoon JH, Hwang J, Son SU, et al. How Can Insulin Resistance Cause Alzheimer's Disease? *Int J Mol Sci*. 2023 Feb 9; 24(4): 3506. doi: 10.3390/ijms24043506.

245 Ouanes S, Popp J. High Cortisol and the Risk of Dementia and Alzheimer's Disease: A Review of the Literature. *Front Aging Neurosci.* 2019 Mar 1; 11: 43. doi: 10.3389/fnagi.2019.00043.

246 Tan ZS, Beiser A, Vasan RS, et al. Thyroid function and the risk of Alzheimer disease: the Framingham Study. *Arch Intern Med.* 2008 Jul 28; 168(14): 1514–1520. doi: 10.1001/archinte.168.14.1514.

247 Zhu X, Zhang C, Feng S, He R, Zhang S. Intestinal microbiota regulates the gut-thyroid axis: the new dawn of improving Hashimoto thyroiditis. *Clin Exp Med.* 2024 Feb 22; 24(1): 39. doi: 10.1007/s10238-024-01304-4.

248 Hara Y, Waters EM, McEwen BS, Morrison JH. Estrogen Effects on Cognitive and Synaptic Health Over the Lifecourse. *Physiol Rev.* 2015 Jul; 95(3): 785–807. doi: 10.1152/physrev.00036.2014.

249 Ellem SJ, Risbridger GP. Aromatase and regulating the estrogen: androgen ratio in the prostate gland. *J Steroid Biochem Mol Biol.* 2010 Feb 28; 118(4–5): 246–251. doi: 10.1016/j.jsbmb.2009.10.015.

250 Hagerman FC, Walsh SJ, Staron RS, et al. Effects of High-Intensity Resistance Training on Untrained Older Men. I. Strength, Cardiovascular, and Metabolic Responses. *Journals of Gerontology, Series A, Biological Sciences and Medical Sciences.* 1 Jul 2000; 55(7): B336–B346. doi: 10.1093/gerona/55.7.B336.

251 Lobo, RA. Hormone-replacement therapy: current thinking. *Nat Rev Endocrinol.* 2017 Apr; 13(4): 220–231. doi: 10.1038/nrendo.2016.164.

252 Wharton W, Baker LD, Gleason CE, et al. Short-term hormone therapy with transdermal estradiol improves cognition for postmenopausal women with Alzheimer's disease: results of a randomized controlled trial. *J Alzheimers Dis.* 2011; 26(3): 495–505. doi: 10.3233/JAD-2011-110341.

253 Yoon B, Chin J, Kim J, et al. Menopausal hormone therapy and mild cognitive impairment: a randomized, placebo-controlled trial. *Menopause.* 2018 Aug; 25(8): 870–876. doi: 10.1097/GME.0000000000001140.

254 Khan I, Saeed K, Jo MG, Kim MO. 17-β Estradiol Rescued Immature Rat Brain against Glutamate-Induced Oxidative Stress and Neurodegeneration via Regulating Nrf2/HO-1 and MAP-Kinase Signaling Pathway. *Antioxidants (Basel).* 2021 Jun 1; 10(6): 892. doi: 10.3390/antiox10060892.

255 Liu JJ, He X, Liu J, Shi JS. Sexual Steroids and Their Receptors Affect Microglia-Mediated Neuroinflammation in Neurodegenerative Diseases. *Biomed J Sci Tech Res.* 2020 Jan; 25(2): 18886–188896. doi: 10.26717/BJSTR.2020.25.004160.

256 Hammond J, Le Q, Goodyer C, Gelfand M, Trifiro M, LeBlanc A. Testosterone-mediated neuroprotection through the androgen receptor in human primary neurons. *J Neurochem.* 2001 Jun; 77(5): 1319–1326. doi: 10.1046/j.1471-4159.2001.00345.x.

257 Azcoitia I, Sierra A, Veiga S, Honda S, Harada N, Garcia-Segura LM. Brain aromatase is neuroprotective. *J Neurobiol.* 2001 Jun 15; 47(4): 318–329. doi: 10.1002/neu.1038.

258 Ma C, Wu X, Shen X, et al. Sex differences in traumatic brain injury: a multi-dimensional exploration in genes, hormones, cells, individuals, and society. *Chin Neurosurg J.* 2019 Oct 4; 5: 24. doi: 10.1186/s41016-019-0173-8.

259 Verdile G, Asih PR, Barron AM, Wahjoepramono EJ, Ittner LM, Martins RN. The impact of luteinizing hormone and testosterone on beta amyloid (Aβ) accumulation: Animal and human clinical studies. *Horm Behav*. 2015 Nov; 76: 81–90. doi: 10.1016/j.yhbeh.2015.05.020.

260 World Health Organization. *Risk Reduction of Cognitive Decline and Dementia: WHO Guidelines*. 2019. https://www.ncbi.nlm.nih.gov/books/NBK542796.

261 Kinno R, Mori Y, Kubota S, et al. High serum high-density lipoprotein-cholesterol is associated with memory function and gyrification of insular and frontal opercular cortex in an elderly memory-clinic population. *Neuroimage Clin*. 2019; 22: 101746. doi: 10.1016/j.nicl.2019.101746.

262 Ward MA, Bendlin BB, McLaren DG, et al. Low HDL Cholesterol is Associated with Lower Gray Matter Volume in Cognitively Healthy Adults. *Front Aging Neurosci*. 2010 Jul 15; 2: 29. doi: 10.3389/fnagi.2010.00029.

263 Bredesen DE. Reversal of cognitive decline: a novel therapeutic program. *Aging*. 2014 Sep; 6(9): 707–717. doi: 10.18632/aging.100690.

264 Sáiz-Vazquez O, Puente-Martínez A, Ubillos-Landa S, Pacheco-Bonrostro J, Santabárbara J. Cholesterol and Alzheimer's Disease Risk: A Meta-Meta-Analysis. *Brain Sci*. 2020 Jun 18; 10(6): 386. doi: 10.3390/brainsci10060386.

265 Hua R, Li C, Ma Y, Zhong B, Xie W. Low levels of low-density lipoprotein cholesterol and cognitive decline. *Science Bulletin*. 2021 Feb; 66(16): 1684–1690. doi: 10.1016/j.scib.2021.02.018.

266 Isaacson RS, Ganzer CA, Hristov H, et al. The Clinical Practice of Risk Reduction for Alzheimer's Disease: A Precision Medicine Approach. *Alzheimers Dement*. 2018; 14(12): 1663–1673. doi: 10.1016/j.jalz.2018.08.004.

267 Bredesen DE. Reversal of cognitive decline: a novel therapeutic program. *Aging*. 2014 Sep; 6(9): 707–717. doi: 10.18632/aging.100690.

268 Gui Y, Zheng H, Cao RY. Foam Cells in Atherosclerosis: Novel Insights Into Its Origins, Consequences, and Molecular Mechanisms. *Front Cardiovasc Med*. 2022 Apr 13; 9: 845942. doi: 10.3389/fcvm.2022.845942.

269 World Health Organization. *Risk Reduction of Cognitive Decline and Dementia: WHO Guidelines*. 2019. https://www.ncbi.nlm.nih.gov/books/NBK542796.

270 Geifman N, Brinton RD, Kennedy RE, Schneider LS, Butte AJ. Evidence for benefit of statins to modify cognitive decline and risk in Alzheimer's disease. *Alzheimer's Research & Therapy*. 2017 Feb 17; 9(1): 10. doi: 10.1186/s13195-017-0237-y.

271 World Health Organization. *Risk Reduction of Cognitive Decline and Dementia: WHO Guidelines*. 2019. https://www.ncbi.nlm.nih.gov/books/NBK542796.

272 Geifman N, Brinton RD, Kennedy RE, Schneider LS, Butte AJ. Evidence for benefit of statins to modify cognitive decline and risk in Alzheimer's disease. *Alzheimers Res Ther*. 2017 Feb 17; 9(1): 10. doi: 10.1186/s13195-017-0237-y.

273 Cholesterol, Lipids, and Treatments, Including Statins. APOE. 2018. Accessed March 25, 2025. https://www.ApoE4.Info/Wiki/Cholesterol,_Lipids_and_Treatments,_including_statins.

274 Perlmutter D. *Brain Maker: The Power of Gut Microbes to Heal and Protect Your Brain—for Life.* Little, Brown Spark; 2015: 49.

275 Konkel L. Phthalates and Autistic Traits: Exploring the Association between Prenatal Exposures and Child Behavior. *Environ Health Perspect.* 2020 Oct; 128(10): 104001. doi: 10.1289/EHP7127.

276 Can All those Chemicals Be Causing My Asthma? Society of Toxicology. Reviewed May 2015. Accessed April 28, 2025. https://www.toxicology.org/pubs/docs/pr/ToxTopics/TT1_Asthma.pdf.

277 Yang SN, Hsieh CC, Kuo HF, et al. The effects of environmental toxins on allergic inflammation. *Allergy Asthma Immunol Res.* 2014 Nov; 6(6): 478–484. doi: 10.4168/aair.2014.6.6.478.

278 Landrigan PJ, Slutsky J. Are Learning Disabilities Linked to Environmental Toxins? Learning Disabilities Worldwide. Accessed March 25, 2025. https://www.ldworldwide.org/environmental-toxins.

279 Sutton P, Woodruff TJ, Perron J, et al. Toxic environmental chemicals: the role of reproductive health professionals in preventing harmful exposures. *Am J Obstet Gynecol.* 2012 Sep; 207(3): 164–173. doi: 10.1016/j.ajog.2012.01.034.

280 Can Environmental Toxins Cause Parkinson's Disease? Johns Hopkins Medicine. Published April 10, 2022. Accessed March 25, 2025. https://www.hopkinsmedicine.org/health/conditions-and-diseases/parkinsons-disease/can-environmental-toxins-cause-parkinson-disease.

281 Yegambaram M, Manivannan B, Beach TG, Halden RU. Role of environmental contaminants in the etiology of Alzheimer's disease: a review. *Curr Alzheimer Res.* 2015; 12(2): 116–146. doi: 10.2174/1567205012666150204121719.

282 Jackson E, Shoemaker R, Larian N, Cassis L. Adipose Tissue as a Site of Toxin Accumulation. *Compr Physiol.* 2017 Sep 12; 7(4): 1085–1135. doi: 10.1002/cphy.c160038. Correction in *Compr Physiol.* 2018 Jul; 8(3): 1251. doi: 10.1002/cphy.cv08i03corr

283 Crinnion WJ. Environmental medicine, part one: the human burden of environmental toxins and their common health effects. *Altern Med Rev.* 2000 Feb; 5(1): 52–63.

284 Cohen A. *Integrative Environmental Medicine.* Oxford University Press; 2017.

285 Oudi ME, Aouni Z, Mazigh C, et al. Homocysteine and markers of inflammation in acute coronary syndrome. *Exp Clin Cardiol.* 2010 Summer; 15(2): e25–e28. PMID: 20631860.

286 Moulton PV, Yang W. Air pollution, oxidative stress, and Alzheimer's disease. *J Environ Public Health.* 2012 Mar 15: 472751. doi: 10.1155/2012/472751.

287 Genc S, Zadeoglulari Z, Fuss SH, Genc K. The adverse effects of air pollution on the nervous system. *J Toxicol.* 2012 19 Feb: 782462. doi: 10.1155/2012/782462.

288 Chen H, Kwong JC, Copes R, et al. Living near major roads and the incidence of dementia, Parkinson's disease, and multiple sclerosis: a population-based cohort study. *Lancet Public Health.* 2017 Feb 18; 389(10070): 718–726. doi: 10.1016/S0140-6736(16)32399-6.

289   Peters R, Ee N, Peters J, Booth A, Mudway I, Anstey KJ. Air Pollution and Dementia: A Systematic Review. *J Alzheimers Dis*. 2019; 70(s1): S145–S163. doi: 10.3233/JAD-180631.

290   Cacciottolo M, Wang X, Driscoll I, et al. Particulate air pollutants, APOE alleles and their contributions to cognitive impairment in older women and to amyloidogenesis in experimental models. *Transl Psychiatry*. 2017; 7: e1022. doi: 10.1038/tp.2016.280.

291   Faul J, Mendes de Leon C, Gao J, et al. Comparison of Particulate Air Pollution From Different Emission Sources and Incident Dementia in the US. *JAMA Intern Med*. 2023 Oct 1; 183(10): 1080–1089. doi: 10.1001/jamainternmed.2023.3300.

292   U.S. Environmental Protection Agency. An introduction to indoor air quality: Nitrogen dioxide EPA. Published 2010. Accessed February 12, 2025. https://www.epa.gov/indoor-air-quality-iaq/nitrogen-dioxides-impact-indoor-air-quality.

293   Wang S, Zhang J, Zeng X, Zeng Y, Wang S, Chen S. Association of traffic-related air pollution with children's neurobehavioral functions in Quanzhou, China. *Environ Health Perspect*. 2009 Oct; 117(10): 1612–1618. doi: 10.1289/ehp.0800023.

294   Morales E, Julvez J, Torrent M, et al. Association of early-life exposure to household gas appliances and indoor nitrogen dioxide with cognition and attention behavior in preschoolers. *Am J Epidemiol*. 2009 Jun 1; 169(11): 1327–1336. doi: 10.1093/aje/kwp067.

295   Liu J, Lewis G. Environmental Toxicity and Poor Cognitive Outcomes in Children and Adults. *J Environ Health*. 2014 Jan–Feb; 76(6): 130–138.

296   Sherrill S. Electromagnetic Frequency: How it Affects our Brain and our Body. *The Sharper Edge*. 2019 Spring.

297   The World Health Organization has classified EMFs as group 2B carcinogens (possibly cancerous) and a 2016 NIH study found an increased occurrence of rare brain tumors (gliomas) and rare heart tumors from exposure to microwave radiation from cell phones. National Toxicology Program. *Encyclopedia of Toxicology*, 3rd ed. Published April 14, 2014. Accessed March 25, 2025. http://www.sciencedirect.com/science/article/pii/B9780123864543010356.

298   Gunnarsson LG, Bodin L. Occupational Exposures and Neurodegenerative Diseases—A Systematic Literature Review and Meta-Analyses. *Int J Environ Res Public Health*. 2019 Jan 26; 16(3): 337. doi: 10.3390/ijerph16030337.

299   Davanipour Z, Tseng CC, Lee PJ, Sobel E. A case-control study of occupational magnetic field exposure and Alzheimer's disease: results from the California Alzheimer's Disease Diagnosis and Treatment Centers. *BMC Neurol*. 2007 Jun 9; 7: 13. doi: 10.1186/1471-2377-7-13.

300   EU 5G Appeal – Scientists warn of potential serious health effects of 5G. *JRS Eco Wireless*. Published May 31, 2019. Accessed March 25, 2025. https://www.jrseco.com/european-union-5g-appeal-scientists-warn-of-potential-serious-health-effects-of-5g.

301   Kim JH, Lee J-K, Kim H-G, Kim K-B, Kim HR. Possible Effects of Radiofrequency Electromagnetic Field Exposure on Central Nerve System. *Biomol Ther (Seoul)*. 2018 Nov 27; 27(3): 265–275. doi: 10.4062/biomolther.2018.152.

302   Braune S, Wrocklage C, Raczek J, Gailus T, Lucking CH. Resting blood pressure increase during exposure to a radio-frequency magnetic field. *Lancet Public Health*. 1998 Jun 20; (351)9119: 1857–1858. doi: 10.1016/S0140-6736(98)24025-6.

303   Wang Z, Wang L, Zheng S, et al. Effects of electromagnetic fields on serum lipids in workers of a power plant. *Environ Sci Pollut Res Int*. 2016 Feb; 23(3): 2495–2504. doi: 10.1007/s11356-015-5500-9.

304   van Wijngaarden E, Savitz DA, Kleckner RC, Cai J, Loomis D. Exposure to electromagnetic fields and suicide among electric utility workers: a nested case-control study. *West J Med*. 2000 Aug; 173(2): 94–100. doi: 10.1136/ewjm.173.2.94.

305   Luo X, Huang X, Luo Z, et al. Electromagnetic field exposure-induced depression features could be alleviated by heat acclimation based on remodeling the gut microbiota. *Ecotoxicol Environ Saf*. 2021 Nov 15; 228: 112980. doi: 10.1016/j.ecoenv.2021.112980.

306   Bagheri Hosseinabadi M, Khanjani N, Ebrahimi MH, Haji B, Abdolahfard M. The effect of chronic exposure to extremely low-frequency electromagnetic fields on sleep quality, stress, depression and anxiety. *Electromagn Biol Med*. 2019; 38(1): 96–101. doi: 10.1080/15368378.2018.1545665.

307   Kashani ZA, Pakzad R, Fakari FR, et al. Electromagnetic fields exposure on fetal and childhood abnormalities: Systematic review and meta-analysis. *Open Med (Wars)*. 2023 May 12; 18(1): 20230697. doi: 10.1515/med-2023-0697.

308   Mihai CT, Rotinberg P, Brinza F, Vochita G. Extremely low-frequency electromagnetic fields cause DNA strand breaks in normal cells. *J Environ Health Sci Eng*. 2014 Jan 8; 12(1): 15. doi: 10.1186/2052-336X-12-15.

309   Pinto I, Bellieni CV. Fetal and Neonatal Effects of EMF. 2012 Sep. doi: 10.13140/2.1.1341.7605.

310   Wahl S, Engelhardt M, Schaupp P, Lappe C, Ivanov IV. The inner clock-Blue light sets the human rhythm. *J Biophotonics*. 2019 Dec; 12(12): e201900102. doi: 10.1002/jbio.201900102.

311   Singh K, Nagaraj A, Yousuf A, Ganta S, Pareek S, Vishnani P. Effect of electromagnetic radiations from mobile phone base stations on general health and salivary function. *J Int Soc Prev Community Dent*. 2016 Jan–Feb; 6(1): 54–59. doi: 10.4103/2231-0762.175413.

312   Schuermann D, Mevissen M. Manmade Electromagnetic Fields and Oxidative Stress—Biological Effects and Consequences for Health. *Int J Mol Sci*. 2021; 22(7): 3772. doi: 10.3390/ijms22073772.

313   Pall ML. Electromagnetic fields act via activation of voltage-gated calcium channels to produce beneficial or adverse effects. *J Cell Mol Med*. 2013 Aug; 17(8): 958–965. doi: 10.1111/jcmm.12088.

314   Luca M, Luca A, Calandra C. The Role of Oxidative Damage in the Pathogenesis and Progression of Alzheimer's Disease and Vascular Dementia. *Oxid Med Cell Longev*. 2015; 2015: 504678. doi: 10.1155/2015/504678.

315   Taheri M, Mortazavi SM, Moradi M, Mansouri S, Hatam GR, Nouri F. Evaluation of the Effect of Radiofrequency Radiation Emitted From Wi-Fi Router and Mobile Phone Simulator on the Antibacterial Susceptibility of Pathogenic Bacteria *Listeria monocytogenes* and *Escherichia coli*. Dose Response. 2017 Jan 23; 15(1): 1559325816688527. doi: 10.1177/1559325816688527.

316 Mortazavi G, Mortazavi SAR, Mehdizadeh AR. "Triple M" Effect: A Proposed Mechanism to Explain Increased Dental Amalgam Microleakage after Exposure to Radiofrequency Electromagnetic Radiation. *J Biomed Phys Eng*. 2018 Mar 1; 8(1): 141–146.

317 Mortazavi G, Mortazavi SM. Increased mercury release from dental amalgam restorations after exposure to electromagnetic fields as a potential hazard for hypersensitive people and pregnant women. *Rev Environ Health*. 2015; 30(4): 287–292. doi: 10.1515/reveh-2015-0017.

318 Kim JY, Kang SW. Relationships between Dietary Intake and Cognitive Function in Healthy Korean Children and Adolescents. *J Lifestyle Med*. 2017 Jan; 7(1): 10–17. doi: 10.15280/jlm.2017.7.1.10.

319 Pase MP, Himali JJ, Beiser AS, et al. Sugar- and artificially-sweetened beverages and the risks of incident stroke and dementia: A prospective cohort study. *Stroke*. 2017 May; 48(5): 1139–1146. doi: 10.1161/STROKEAHA.116.016027.

320 Choudhary AK, Lee YY. Neurophysiological symptoms and aspartame: What is the connection? *Nutr Neurosci*. 2018 Jun; 21(5): 306–316. doi: 10.1080/1028415X.2017.1288340.

321 Lindseth GN, Coolahan SE, Petros TV, Lindseth PD. Neurobehavioral effects of aspartame consumption. *Res Nurs Health*. 2014 Jun; 37(3): 185–193. doi: 10.1002/nur.21595.

322 Parson RB, Waring RH, Ramsden DB, Williams AC. In vitro effect of the cysteine metabolites homocysteic acid, homocysteine and cysteic acid upon human neuronal cell lines. *Neurotoxicology*. 1998 Aug–Oct; 19(4–5): 599–603.

323 Jianqin S, Leiming X, Lu X, Yelland GW, Ni J, Clarke AJ. Effects of milk containing only A2 beta casein versus milk containing both A1 and A2 beta casein proteins on gastrointestinal physiology, symptoms of discomfort, and cognitive behavior of people with self-reported intolerance to traditional cows' milk. *Nutr J*. 2016 Apr 2; 15: 35. doi: 10.1186/s12937-016-0147-z.

324 Niaz K, Zaplatic E, Spoor J. Extensive use of monosodium glutamate: A threat to public health? *EXCLI J*. 2018 Mar 19; 17: 273–278. doi: 10.17179/excli2018-1092.

325 McCann D, Barrett A, Cooper A, et al. Food additives and hyperactive behaviour in 3-year-old and 8/9-year-old children in the community: a randomised, double-blinded, placebo-controlled trial. *Lancet Public Health*. 2007 Nov 3; 370(9598): 1560–1507. doi: 10.1016/S0140-6736(07)61306-3.

326 Novembre E, Dini L, Bernardini R, Resti M, Vierucci A. Unusual reactions to food additives. *Pediatr Med Chir Med Surg Pediatrics*. 1992; 14: 39–42.

327 Elhkim MO, Héraud F, Bemrah N, et al. New considerations regarding the risk assessment on Tartrazine: An update toxicological assessment, intolerance reactions and maximum theoretical daily intake in France. *Regul Toxicol Pharmacol*. 2007 Apr; 47(3): 308–316. doi: 10.1016/j.yrtph.2006.11.004.

328 Sasaki YF, Kawaguchi S, Kamaya A, et al. The comet assay with 8 mouse organs: results with 39 currently used food additives. *Mutat Res*. 2002 Aug 26; 519(1–2): 103–119. doi: 10.1016/s1383-5718(02)00128-6.

329 Merinas-Amo R, Martínez-Jurado M, Jurado-Güeto S, Alonso-Moraga Á, Merinas-Amo T. Biological Effects of Food Coloring in In Vivo and In Vitro Model Systems. *Foods*. 2019 May 24; 8(5): 176. doi: 10.1016/j.yrtph.2006.11.004.

330 Weiss B. The intersection of neurotoxicology and endocrine disruption. *Neurotoxicology*. 2012; 33(6): 1410–1419. doi: 10.1016/j.neuro.2012.05.014.

331 Guerrero-Bosagna C, Skinner MK. Environmentally induced epigenetic transgenerational inheritance of phenotype and disease. *Mol Cell Endocrinol*. 2012 May 6; 354(1-2): 3–8. doi: 10.1016/j.mce.2011.10.004.

332 Examples are: di(2-ethylhexyl)phthalate (DEHP), diisononyl phthalate (DINP), diisodecyl phthalate (DIDP), dimethyl phthalate (DMP), diethyl phthalate (DEP), and dibutyl phthalate (DPB).

333 Zhang Q, Chen XZ, Huang X, Wang M, Wu J. The association between prenatal exposure to phthalates and cognition and neurobehavior of children-evidence from birth cohorts. *Neurotoxicology*. 2019 Jul; 73: 199–212. doi: 10.1016/j.neuro.2019.04.007.

334 Bornehag C, Lindh C, Reichenberg A, et al. Association of Prenatal Phthalate Exposure With Language Development in Early Childhood. *JAMA Pediatr*. 2018; 172(12): 1169–1176. doi:10.1001/jamapediatrics.2018.3115.

335 Wang Y, Qian H. Phthalates and Their Impacts on Human Health. *Healthcare (Basel)*. 2021 May 18; 9(5): 603. doi: 10.3390/healthcare9050603.

336 Zhou F, Jin Z, Zhu L, Huang F, Ye A, Hou C. A preliminary study on the relationship between environmental endocrine disruptors and precocious puberty in girls. *J Pediatr Endocrinol Metab*. 2022 Jun 14; 35(8): 989–997. doi: 10.1515/jpem-2021-0691.

337 Weng X, Tan Y, Fei Q, et al. Association between mixed exposure of phthalates and cognitive function among the U.S. elderly from NHANES 2011-2014: Three statistical models. *Sci Total Environ*. 2022 Jul 1; 828: 154362. doi: 10.1016/j.scitotenv.2022.154362.

338 Guillette EA, Meza MM, Aquilar MG, Soto AD, Enedina I. An anthropological approach to the evaluation of preschool children exposed to pesticides in Mexico. *Environ Health Perspect*. 1998; 106: 347–353. doi: 10.1289/ehp.98106347.

339 Yan D, Zhang Y, Liu L, Yan H. Pesticide exposure and risk of Alzheimer's disease: a systematic review and meta-analysis. *Sci Rep*. 2016 Sep 1; 6: 32222. doi: 10.1038/srep32222.

340 Weisenburger DD. A Review and Update with Perspective of Evidence that the Herbicide Glyphosate (Roundup) is a Cause of Non-Hodgkin Lymphoma. *Clin Lymphoma Myeloma Leuk*. 2021 Sep; 21(9): 621–630. doi: 10.1016/j.clml.2021.04.009.

341 Peillex C, Pelletier M. The impact and toxicity of glyphosate and glyphosate-based herbicides on health and immunity. *J Immunotoxicol*. 2020 Dec; 17(1): 163–174. doi: 10.1080/1547691X.2020.1804492.

342 Winstone JK, Pathak KV, Winslow W, et al. Glyphosate infiltrates the brain and increases pro-inflammatory cytokine TNFα: implications for neurodegenerative disorders. *J Neuroinflammation*. 2022 Jul 28; 19(1): 193. doi: 10.1186/s12974-022-02544-5.

343 Seneff S. *Toxic Legacy*. Chelsea Green Publishing; 2021: 18.

344 Honda T, Ohara T, Shinohara M, et al. Serum elaidic acid concentration and risk of dementia: The Hisayama Study. *Neurology*. 2019 Nov 26; 93(22): e2053–e2064. doi: 10.1212/WNL.0000000000008464.

345 Jiang H, Justice LM, Purtell KM, Bates R. Exposure to Environmental Toxicants and Early Language Development for Children Reared in Low-Income Households. *Clin Pediatr (Phila)*. 2020 Jun; 59(6): 557–565. doi: 10.1177/0009922820908591.

346 Bai J, Wang Y, Deng S, Yang Y, Chen S, Wu Z. Microplastics caused embryonic growth retardation and placental dysfunction in pregnant mice by activating GRP78/IRE1α/JNK axis induced apoptosis and endoplasmic reticulum stress. *Part Fibre Toxicol*. 2024 Sep 11; 21(1): 36. doi: 10.1186/s12989-024-00595-5; Riesgo VR, Sellinger EP, Brinks AS, Juraska JM, Willing J. Effects of maternal LPS and developmental exposure to an environmentally relevant phthalate mixture on neuron number in the rat medial prefrontal cortex. *Neurotoxicol Teratol*. 2024 Jul-Aug; 04(2024). doi: 10.1016/j.ntt.2024.107370.

347 Volatile Organic Compounds' Impact on Indoor Air Quality. EPA. Updated August 13, 2024. Accessed March 25, 2025. https://www.epa.gov/indoor-air-quality-iaq/volatile-organic-compounds-impact-indoor-air-quality.

348 Lu Z, Li CM, Qiao Y, Yan Y, Yang X. Effect of inhaled formaldehyde on learning and memory of mice. *Indoor Air*. 2008 Apr; 18(2): 77–83. doi: 10.1111/j.1600-0668.2008.00524.x.

349 Wang S, Zhang J, Zeng X, Zeng Y, Wang S, Chen S. Association of traffic-related air pollution with children's neurobehavioral functions in Quanzhou, China. *Environ Health Perspect*. 2009; 117(10): 1612–1618. doi: 10.1289/ehp.0800023.

350 Suglia SF, Gryparis A, Wright RO, Schwartz J, Wright RJ. Association of black carbon and cognition among children in a prospective birth cohort study. *Am J Epidemiol*. 2008; 167(3): 280–286. doi: 10.1093/aje/kwm308.

351 Krishnamoorthy Y, Sarveswaran G, Sivaranjini K, Sakthivel M, Majella MG, Kumar SG. Association between Indoor Air Pollution and Cognitive Impairment among Adults in Rural Puducherry, South India. *J Neurosci Rural Pract*. 2018 Oct-Dec; 9(4): 529–534. doi: 10.4103/jnrp.jnrp_123_18.

352 Balwierz R, Biernat P, Jasińska-Balwierz A, et al. Potential Carcinogens in Makeup Cosmetics. *Int J Environ Res Public Health*. 2023 Mar 8; 20(6): 4780. doi: 10.3390/ijerph20064780.

353 Goldberg M, Chang CJ, Ogunsina K, et al. Personal Care Product Use during Puberty and Incident Breast Cancer among Black, Hispanic/Latina, and White Women in a Prospective US-Wide Cohort. *Environ Health Perspect*. 2024 Feb; 132(2): 27001. doi: 10.1289/EHP13882.

354 Zlatnik MG. Endocrine-Disrupting Chemicals and Reproductive Health. *J Midwifery Women's Health*. 2016 Jul; 61(4): 442–455. doi: 10.1111/jmwh.12500.

355 Ullah S, Ahmad S, Guo X, et al. A review of the endocrine disrupting effects of micro and nano plastic and their associated chemicals in mammals. *Front Endocrinol (Lausanne)*. 2023 Jan 16; 13: 1084236. doi: 10.3389/fendo.2022.

356 Campanale C, Massarelli C, Savino I, Locaputo V, Uricchio VF. A Detailed Review Study on Potential Effects of Microplastics and Additives of Concern on Human Health. *Int J Environ Res Public Health*. 2020 Feb 13; 17(4): 1212. doi: 10.3390/ijerph17041212.

357 Choi G, Keil AP, Richardson DB, et al. Pregnancy exposure to organophosphate esters and the risk of attention-deficit hyperactivity disorder in the Norwegian mother, father and child cohort study. *Environ Int*. 2021 Sep; 154: 106549. doi: 10.1016/j.envint.2021.106549.

358 Gaspar L, Bartman S, Coppotelli G, Ross JM. Acute Exposure to Microplastics Induced Changes in Behavior and Inflammation in Young and Old Mice. *Int J Mol Sci*. 2023 Aug 1; 24(15): 12308. doi: 10.3390/ijms241512308.

359 Garcia MM, Romero AS, Merkley SD, et al. *In Vivo* Tissue Distribution of Polystyrene or Mixed Polymer Microspheres and Metabolomic Analysis after Oral Exposure in Mice. *Env Health Perspectives*. 132(4): 47005. doi: 10.1289/EHP134.

360 Pasquini E, Ferrante F, Passaponti L, Pavone FS, Costantini I, Baracchi D. Microplastics reach the brain and interfere with honey bee cognition. *Sci Total Environ*. 2024 Feb 20; 912: 169362. doi: 10.1016/j.scitotenv.2023.169362.

361 Tamargo A, Molinero N, Reinosa JJ, et al. PET microplastics affect human gut microbiota communities during simulated gastrointestinal digestion, first evidence of plausible polymer biodegradation during human digestion. *Sci Rep*. 2022; 12: 528. doi: 10.1038/s41598-021-04489-w.

362 Bozkurt HS, Yörüklü HC, Bozkurt K, et al. Biodegradation of microplastic by probiotic bifidobacterium. *Int J Glob*.Warm? 2022; 26(4). doi: 10.1504/IJGW.2022.122435.

363 Li N, Wang J, Liu P, Li J, Xu C. Multi-omics reveals that Bifidobacterium breve M-16V may alleviate the immune dysregulation caused by nanopolystyrene. *Environ Int*. 2022 May; 163: 107191. doi: 10.1016/j.envint.2022.107191.

364 Types of Drinking Water Contaminants. EPA. Updated August 17, 2024. Accessed March 25, 2025. https://www.epa.gov/ccl/types-drinking-water-contaminants.

365 Perfluoroalkyl and Polyfluoroalkyl Substances (PFAS). National Institute of Environmental Health Sciences. Updated March 6, 2025. Accessed March 25, 2025. https://www.niehs.nih.gov/health/topics/agents/pfc.

366 Fenton SE, Ducatman A, Boobis A, et al. Per- and Polyfluoroalkyl Substance Toxicity and Human Health Review: Current State of Knowledge and Strategies for Informing Future Research. *Environ Toxicol Chem*. 2021 Mar; 40(3): 606–630. doi: 10.1002/etc.4890.

367 Indoor HEPA filters significantly reduce pollution indoors when outside air unhealthy, study finds. *ScienceDaily*. Published September 25, 2018. Accessed March 25, 2025. http://www.sciencedaily.com/releases/2018/09/180925110030.htm.

368 Let the Air in. American Lung Association. Published August 31, 2023. Accessed March 25, 2025. https://www.lung.org/blog/indoor-air-quality-improvements.

369 Ramnarace, C. Do "Green" Cleaners Work? *AARP Bulletin*. 2011 March 14.

370 Opalchenova G, Obreshkova D. Comparative studies on the activity of basil — an essential oil from *Ocimum basilicum* L. — against multidrug resistant clinical isolates of the genera *Staphylococcus*, *Enterococcus* and *Pseudomonas* by using different test methods. *J Microbiol Methods*. 2003 Jul; 54(1): 105-110. doi: 10.1016/s0167-7012(03)00012-5.

371 National Research Council (US) Subcommittee on Immunotoxicology. The Capacity of Toxic Agents to Compromise the Immune System (Biologic Markers of Immunosuppression). In *Biologic Markers in Immunotoxicology*. Washington DC: National Academies Press; 1992. https://www.ncbi.nlm.nih.gov/books/NBK235670.

372 Balali-Mood M, Naseri K, Tahergorabi Z, Khazdair MR, Sadeghi M. Toxic Mechanisms of Five Heavy Metals: Mercury, Lead, Chromium, Cadmium, and Arsenic. *Front Pharmacol*. 2021 Apr 13; 12: 643972. doi: 10.3389/fphar.2021.643972.

373 Yıldız S, Gözü Pirinççioğlu A, Arıca E. Evaluation of Heavy Metal (Lead, Mercury, Cadmium, and Manganese) Levels in Blood, Plasma, and Urine of Adolescents With Aggressive Behavior. *Cureus*. 2023 Jan 17; 15(1): e33902. doi: 10.7759/cureus.33902.

374 Gennings C, Ellis R, Ritter JK. Linking empirical estimates of body burden of environmental chemicals and wellness using NHANES data. *Environ Int*. 2012 Feb; 39(1): 56-65. doi: 10.1016/j.envint.2011.09.002.

375 Miranda ML, Kim D, Galeano MA, Paul CJ, Hull AP, Morgan SP. The relationship between early childhood blood lead levels and performance on end-of-grade tests. *Environ Health Perspect*. 2007 Aug; 115(8): 1242-1247. doi: 10.1289/ehp.9994.

376 'Crisis mode': Flint kids' reading level falls 75% since lead contamination. RT International. Published February 7, 2018. Accessed March 25, 2025. https://www.rt.com/usa/418159-flint-reading-levels-water-lead.

377 Shih RA, Hu H, Weisskopf MG, Schwartz BS. Cumulative lead dose and cognitive function in adults: A review of studies that measured both blood lead and bone lead. *Environ Health Perspect*. 2007; 115(3): 483-492. doi: 10.1289/ehp.9786.

378 The Toxic Truth: Children's Exposure to Lead Pollution Undermines a Generation of Future Potential. UNICEF. Published 2020. Accessed March 25, 2025. https://www.unicef.org/sites/default/files/2020-07/The-toxic-truth-children%E2%80%99s-exposure-to-lead-pollution-2020.pdf.

379 Weuve J, Korrick SA, Weisskopf MG, et al. Cumulative exposure to lead in relation to cognitive function in older women. *Environ Health Perspect*. 2009; 117(4): 574-580. doi: 10.1289/ehp.11846.

380 Stewart WF, Schwartz BS. Effects of lead on the adult brain: A 15-year exploration. *Am J Ind Med*. 2007; 50(10): 729-739. doi: 10.1002/ajim.20434.

381 Mahaffey KR, Clickner RP, Bodurow CC. Blood organic mercury and dietary mercury intake: National Health and Nutrition Examination Survey, 1999 and 2000. *Environ Health Perspect*. 2004 Apr; 112(5): 562-570. doi: 10.1289/ehp.6587; Mahaffey KR. U.S. EPA, "Methylmercury Epidemiology Update," Slide #9 of presentation given at the National Forum on Contaminants in Fish, San Diego, January 2004.

382 Ynalvez R, Gutierrez J, Gonzalez-Cantu H. Mini-review: toxicity of mercury as a consequence of enzyme alteration. *Biometals*. 2016 Oct; 29(5): 781-788. doi: 10.1007/s10534-016-9967-8.

383 da Silva DCB, Bittencourt LO, Baia-da-Silva DC, et al. Methylmercury Causes Neurodegeneration and Downregulation of Myelin Basic Protein in the Spinal Cord of Offspring Rats after Maternal Exposure. *Int J Mol Sci*. 2022 Mar 29; 23(7): 3777. doi: 10.3390/ijms23073777.

384 Moneim AE. Mercury-induced neurotoxicity and neuroprotective effects of berberine. *Neural Regen Res*. 2015 Jun; 10(6): 881–882. doi: 10.4103/1673-5374.158336.

385 Khangura SD, Seal K, Esfandiari S, et al. Appendix 20, Historical Overview of the Amalgam Debate. In Composite Resin Versus Amalgam for Dental Restorations: A Health Technology Assessment [Internet]. Ottawa (ON): Canadian Agency for Drugs and Technologies in Health; 2018 Mar. (Health Technology Assessment Report, No. 147.) Accessed March 25, 2025. https://www.ncbi.nlm.nih.gov/books/NBK531943.

386 Cleaner Power Plants. EPA. Published June 10, 2016. Accessed March 25, 2025. https://19january2017snapshot.epa.gov/mats/cleaner-power-plants_.html.

387 National Wildlife Federation. Mercury Pollution from Coal-fired Power Plants Fact Sheet. Published March 2011. Accessed March 25, 2025. https://www.nwf.org/~/media/PDFs/Global-Warming/NWF-Mercury-Power-Plant-Factsheet_March2011.ashx.

388 What you need to know about mercury in fish and shellfish. Food and Drug Administration. Published March 2004. Accessed March 25, 2025. https://www.fda.gov/food/environmental-contaminants-food/fdaepa-2004-advice-what-you-need-know-about-mercury-fish-and-shellfish.

389 Alzheimer's Disease and Mercury Induced Dementia. IAOMT. Accessed March 25, 2025. http://iaomt.org/wp-content/uploads/infogfx-mercury-induced-dementia-v02.jpg.

390 Rahimzadeh MR, Rahimzadeh MR, Kazemi S, Amiri RJ, Pirzadeh M, Moghadamnia AA. Aluminum Poisoning with Emphasis on Its Mechanism and Treatment of Intoxication. *Emerg Med Int*. 2022 Jan 11; 2022: 1480553. doi: 10.1155/2022/1480553.

391 Jaishankar M, Tseten T, Anbalagan N, et al. Toxicity, mechanism and health effects of some heavy metals. *Interdiscip Toxicol*. 2014 Jun; 7(2): 60–72. doi: 10.2478/intox-2014-0009.

392 WHO-Joint FAO/WHO Expert Committee on Food Additives—Summary Report. July 4, 2011.

393 Wang L. Entry and Deposit of Aluminum in the Brain. *Adv Exp Med Biol*. 2018; 1091: 39–51. doi: 10.1007/978-981-13-1370-7_3.

394 Crouse DC. *Prevent Alzheimer's, Autism and Stroke*. Etiological Publishing; 2016: 34.

395 Mirza A, King A, Troakes C, Exley C. Aluminum in Brain Tissue in Familial Alzheimer's Disease (preprint). *J Trace Elem Med Biol*. 2017 Mar; 40: 30–36. doi: 10.1016/j.jtemb.2016.12.001.

396 Virk SA, Eslick GD. Aluminum Levels in Brain, Serum, and Cerebrospinal Fluid Are Higher in Alzheimer's Disease Cases than in Controls. A series of meta-analyses. *J Alzheimers Disease*. 2015; 47(3): 629–638. doi: 10.3233/JAD-150193.

397 Shimizu H, Mori T, Koyama M, et al. A Correlative Study of the Aluminum Content and Aging Changes of the Brain in Non-Demented Elderly Subjects. *Nihon Ronen Igakkai Zasshi*. 1994 Dec 31; 12: 950–960. doi: 10.3143/geriatrics.31.950.

398   Arsenic and Cancer Risk. American Cancer Society. Updated June 1, 2023. Accessed March 25, 2025. https://www.cancer.org/cancer/risk-prevention/chemicals/arsenic.html.

399   Jaishankar M, Tseten T, Anbalagan N, et al. Toxicity, mechanism and health effects of some heavy metals. *Interdiscip Toxicol*. 2014 Jun; 7(2): 60–72. doi: 10.2478/intox-2014-0009.

400   Sartori AC, Vance DE, Slater LZ, Crowe M. The impact of inflammation on cognitive function in older adults: implications for healthcare practice and research. *J Neurosci Nurs*. 2012 Aug; 44(4): 206–217. doi: 10.1097/JNN.0b013e3182527690.

401   Xie J, Van Hoecke L, Vandenbroucke RE. The Impact of Systemic Inflammation on Alzheimer's Disease Pathology. *Front Immunol*. 2022 Jan; 12: 796867. doi: 10.3389/fimmu.2021.796867.

402   Walker KA, Windham BG, Power MC, et al. The association of mid- to late-life systemic inflammation with white matter structure in older adults: The Atherosclerosis Risk in Communities Study. *Neurobiol Aging*. 2018 Aug; 68: 26–33. doi: 10.1016/j.neurobiolaging.2018.03.031.

403   Nehring SM, Goyal A, Patel BC. C Reactive Protein. StatPearls. Published January 2024. Accessed March 25, 2025. https://www.ncbi.nlm.nih.gov/books/NBK441843.

404   Coelho GDP, Ayres LFA, Barreto DS, Henriques BD, Prado MRMC, Passos CMD. Acquisition of microbiota according to the type of birth: an integrative review. *Rev Lat Am Enfermagem*. 2021 Jul 19; 29: e3446. doi: 10.1590/1518.8345.4466.3446.

405   Fouquier J, Moreno Huizar N, Donnelly J, et al. The Gut Microbiome in Autism: Study-Site Effects and Longitudinal Analysis of Behavior Change. *mSystems*. 2021 Apr 6; 6(2): e00848–20. doi: 10.1128/mSystems.00848-20.

406   Checa-Ros A, Jeréz-Calero A, Molina-Carballo A, Campoy C, Muñoz-Hoyos A. Current Evidence on the Role of the Gut Microbiome in ADHD Pathophysiology and Therapeutic Implications. *Nutrients*. 2021 Jan 16; 13(1): 249. doi: 10.3390/nu13010249.

407   Aleman RS, Moncada M, Aryana KJ. Leaky Gut and the Ingredients That Help Treat It: A Review. *Molecules*. 2023 Jan 7; 28(2): 619. doi: 10.3390/molecules28020619.

408   Signs and Symptoms of Untreated Lyme Disease. Centers for Disease Control and Prevention. Accessed March 25, 2025. https://www.cdc.gov/lyme/signs-symptoms/index.html.

409   The CDC Reveals the Truth About Lyme Disease. Amen Clinics. Published November 15, 2022. Accessed March 25, 2025. https://www.amenclinics.com/blog/the-cdc-reveals-the-truth-about-lyme-disease.

410   Notice to Readers Recommendations for Test Performance and Interpretation from the Second National Conference on Serologic Diagnosis of Lyme Disease. Centers for Disease Control and Prevention. Published August 11, 1995. Accessed March 25, 2025. https://www.cdc.gov/mmwr/preview/mmwrhtml/00038469.htm.

411   Harding CF, Pytte CL, Page KG, et al. Mold inhalation causes innate immune activation, neural, cognitive and emotional dysfunction. *Brain Behav Immun*. 2020 Jul; 87: 218–228. doi: 10.1016/j.bbi.2019.11.006.

412 Li X, Kolltveit KM, Tronstad L, Olsen I. Systemic Diseases Caused by Oral Infection. *Clin Microbiol Rev*. 2000; 13. doi: 10.1128/cmr.13.4.547.

413 Hasturk H, Kantarci A, Van Dyke TE. Oral inflammatory diseases and systemic inflammation: role of the macrophage. *Front Immunol*. 2012 May 16; 3: 118. doi: 10.3389/fimmu.2012.00118.

414 Si J, Lee C, Ko G. Oral Microbiota: Microbial Biomarkers of Metabolic Syndrome Independent of Host Genetic Factors. *Front Cell Infect Microbiol*. 2017 Dec 15; 7: 516. doi: 10.3389/fcimb.2017.00516.

415 Watanabe K, Katagiri S, Takahashi H, et al. Porphyromonas gingivalis impairs glucose uptake in skeletal muscle associated with altering gut microbiota. *FASEB J*. 2021 Feb; 35(2): e21171. doi: 10.1096/fj.202001158R.

416 Yang Y, Cai Q, Zheng W, et al. Oral microbiome and obesity in a large study of low-income and African-American populations. *J Oral Microbiol*. 2019; 11: 1650597. doi: 10.1080/20002297.2019.1650597.

417 Goodson JM, Groppo D, Halem S, Carpino E. Is Obesity an Oral Bacterial Disease? *Journal of Dental Research*. 2009 Jul 8. doi: 10.1177/0022034509338353.

418 Latti BR, Kalburge JV, Birajdar SB, Latti RG. Evaluation of relationship between dental caries, diabetes mellitus and oral microbiota in diabetics. *J Oral Maxillofac Pathol*. 2018 May–Aug; 22(2): 282. doi: 10.4103/jomfp.JOMFP_163_16.

419 Preshaw PM, Alba AL, Herrera D, et al. Periodontitis and diabetes: a two-way relationship. *Diabetologia*. 2012 Jan; 55(1): 21–31. doi: 10.1007/s00125-011-2342-y.

420 Tonomura S, Ihara M, Kawano T, et al. Intracerebral hemorrhage and deep microbleeds associated with cnm-positive Streptococcus mutans; a hospital cohort study. *Scientific Reports*. 2016 Feb 5. doi: 10.1038/srep20074.

421 Patrakka O, Pienimäki JP, Tuomisto S, et al. Oral Bacterial Signatures in Cerebral Thrombi of Patients With Acute Ischemic Stroke Treated With Thrombectomy. *J Am Heart Assoc*. 2019 Jun 4; 8(11): e012330. doi: 10.1161/JAHA.119.012330.

422 Kim J, Amar S. Periodontal disease and systemic conditions: a bidirectional relationship. *Odontology*. 2006 Sep; 94(1): 10–21. doi: 10.1007/s10266-006-0060-6.

423 Esfahanian V, Shamami Mehrnaz S, Shamami Mehrnoosh S. Relationship between osteoporosis and periodontal disease: review of the literature. *J Dentistry (Iran)*. 2012; 9(4): 256–264.

424 Scher JU, Sczesnak A, Longman RS, et al. Expansion of intestinal Prevotella copri correlates with enhanced susceptibility to arthritis. *Elife*. 2013 Nov 5; 2: e01202. doi: 10.7554/eLife.01202.

425 Poor dental health may lead to Alzheimer's. Journal of Alzheimer's Disease. Published July 30, 2013. Accessed March 25, 2025. https://www.j-alz.com/content/poor-dental-health-may-lead-alzheimers.

426 Liu S, Dashper SG, Zhao R. Association Between Oral Bacteria and Alzheimer's Disease: A Systematic Review and Meta-Analysis. *J Alzheimers Dis*. 2023; 91(1): 129–150. doi: 10.3233/JAD-220627.

427 U.S. Department of Health and Human Services. Oral Health in America: A Report of the Surgeon General. U.S. Department of Health and Human Services, National Institute of Dental and Craniofacial Research, National Institutes of Health, 2000.

428 Eke PI, Wei L, Borgnakke WS, et al. Periodontitis prevalence in adults ≥ 65 years of age, in the USA. *Periodontol 2000*. 2016 Oct; 72(1): 76–95. doi: 10.1111/prd.12145.

429 About Periodontal (Gum) Disease. Centers for Disease Control and Prevention. Published May 15, 2024. Accessed March 25, 2025. https://www.cdc.gov/oralhealth/conditions/periodontal-disease.html.

430 Putt MS, Mallatt ME, Messmann LL, Proskin HM. A 6-month clinical investigation of custom tray application of peroxide gel with or without doxycycline as adjuncts to scaling and root planing for treatment of periodontitis. *Am J Dent*. 2014 Oct; 27(5): 273–284. PMID: 25842461.

431 Dagli N, Dagli R, Mahmoud RS, Baroudi K. Essential oils, their therapeutic properties, and implication in dentistry: A review. *J Int Soc Prev Community Dent*. 2015 Sep–Oct; 5(5): 335–40. doi: 10.4103/2231-0762.165933.

432 Thosar N, Basak S, Bahadure RN, Rajurkar M. Antimicrobial efficacy of five essential oils against oral pathogens: An in vitro study. *Eur J Dent*. 2013 Sep; 7(Suppl 1): S071–S077. doi: 10.4103/1305-7456.119078.

433 Morozumi T, Kubota T, Abe D, Shimizu T, Nohno K, Yoshie H. Microbiological effect of essential oils in combination with subgingival ultrasonic instrumentation and mouth rinsing in chronic periodontitis patients. *Int J Dent*. 2013; 146479. doi: 10.1155/2013/146479.

434 Debelian GJ, Olsen I, Tronstad L. Anaerobic Bacteremia and Fungemia in Patients Undergoing Endodontic Therapy: An Overview. *Ann Periodontol*. 01 Jul 1998; 3(1): 281–287. doi: 10.1902/annals.1998.3.1.281.

435 Davis DR. Declining Fruit and Vegetable Nutrient Composition: What Is the Evidence? *HortScience*. 2009; 44(1): 15–19. doi: 10.21273/HORTSCI.44.1.15.

436 Rynfield R. Nutrient Depletion of U.S. Farmlands and Soil: A Critical Review. *J Am Center Nutr*. 2022; 1(1): 19–20.

437 Nutritional Deficiencies Due to Soil Depletion and the Necessity of Supplements. Pharmaden. Published November 2013. Accessed March 25, 2025. https://www.pharmaden.net/wp-content/uploads/2013/11/pharmaden-reasearch.pdf.

438 Dietrich T, Joshipura KJ, Dawson-Hughes B, Bischoff-Ferrari HA. Association between serum concentrations of 25-hydroxyvitamin D3 and periodontal disease in the US population. *Am J Clin Nutr*. 2004 Jul; 80(1): 108–113. doi: 10.1093/ajcn/80.1.108.

439 Rossi M, Bosetti C, Negri E, Lagiou P, La Vecchia C. Flavonoids, proanthocyanidins, and cancer risk: a network of case-control studies from Italy. *Nutr Cancer*. 2010; 62(7): 871–877. doi: 10.1080/01635581.2010.509534.

440 Rasmussen SE, Frederiksen H, Struntze Krogholm K, Poulsen L. Dietary proanthocyanidins: occurrence, dietary intake, bioavailability, and protection against cardiovascular disease. *Mol Nutr Food Res*. 2005 Feb; 49(2): 159–174. doi: 10.1002/mnfr.200400082.

441 Unusan N. Proanthocyanidins in grape seeds: An updated review of their health benefits and potential uses in the food industry. *J Funct Foods*. 2020 Apr; 67: 103861. doi.org/10.1016/j.jff.2020.103861.

442 Exercise, Eating Right, Watching Weight Benefit Oral Health. *J Am Dent Assoc*. 2005 Oct 1; 136(10): 1370. doi: 10.14219/jada.archive.2005.0043.

443 Balogun SA, Philbrick JT. Delirium, a Symptom of UTI in the Elderly: Fact or Fable? A Systematic Review. *Can Geriatr J*. 2014 Mar; 17(1): 22–26. doi: 10.5770/cgj.17.90.

444 For more pro-inflammatory and anti-inflammatory foods, see ellwoodthompsons.com, verywellmind.com, amenclinics.com, webmd.com/diet/anti-inflammatory-diet-road-to-good-health, health.harvard.edu/staying-healthy/foods-that-fight-inflammation, hopkinsmedicine.org/health/wellness-and-prevention/anti-inflammatory-diet.

445 Gupta SC, Patchva S, Aggarwal BB. Therapeutic roles of curcumin: lessons learned from clinical trials. AAPS J. 2013 Jan; 15(1): 195–218. doi: 10.1208/s12248-012-9432-8..

446 Kunnumakkara AB, Sailo BL, Banik K, et al. Chronic diseases, inflammation, and spices: how are they linked? *J Transl Med*. 2018 Jan 25; 16(1): 14. doi: 10.1186/s12967-018-1381-2.

447 Gray SL, Anderson ML, Dublin S, et al. Cumulative use of strong anticholinergics and incident dementia: a prospective cohort study. *JAMA Intern Med*. 2015 Mar; 175(3): 401–407. doi: 10.1001/jamainternmed.2014.7663.

448 Billioti de Gage S, Moride Y, Ducruet T, et al. Benzodiazepine use and risk of Alzheimer's disease: case-control study. *BMJ*. 2014; 349. doi: 10.1136/bmj.g5205.

449 Billioti de Gage S, Moride Y, Ducruet T, et al. Benzodiazepine use and risk of Alzheimer's disease: case-control study. *BMJ*. 2014; 349. doi: 10.1136/bmj.g5205.

450 Billioti de Gage S, Bégaud B, Bazin F, et al. Benzodiazepine use and risk of dementia: prospective population based study. *BMJ*. 2012 Sep 27; 345: e6231. doi: 10.1136/bmj.e6231.

451 Solomon A, Kivipelto M, Wolozin B, Zhou J, Whitmer RA. Midlife Serum Cholesterol and Increased Risk of Alzheimer's and Vascular Dementia Three Decades Later. *Dement Geriatr Cogn Disord*. 2009; 28: 75–80. doi: 10.1159/000231980.

452 Elias PK, Elias MF, D'Agostino RB, Sullivan LM, Wolf PA. Serum Cholesterol and Cognitive Performance in the Framingham Heart Study. *Psychosom Med*. 2005; 67: 24–30. doi: 10.1097/01.psy.0000151745.67285.c2.

453 Jin U, Park SJ, Park SM. Cholesterol Metabolism in the Brain and Its Association with Parkinson's Disease. *Exp Neurobiol*. 2019 Oct 31; 28(5): 554–567. doi: 10.5607/en.2019.28.5.554.

454 Zhang J, Liu Q. Cholesterol metabolism and homeostasis in the brain. *Protein Cell*. 2015 Apr; 6(4): 254–264. doi: 10.1007/s13238-014-0131-3.

455 Pang K, Liu C, Tong J, Ouyang W, Hu S, Tang Y. Higher Total Cholesterol Concentration May Be Associated with Better Cognitive Performance among Elderly Females. *Nutrients*. 2022 Oct 9; 14(19): 4198. doi: 10.3390/nu14194198.

456 Lee J, Lee S, Min JY, Min KB. Association between Serum Lipid Parameters and Cognitive Performance in Older Adults. *J Clin Med*. 2021 Nov 19; 10(22): 5405. doi: 10.3390/jcm10225405.

457 van Vliet P, van de Water W, de Craen AJ, Westendorp RG. The influence of age on the association between cholesterol and cognitive function. *Exp Gerontol*. 2009 Jan–Feb; 44(1-2): 112–122. doi: 10.1016/j.exger.2008.05.004.

458 van Vliet P. Cholesterol and late-life cognitive decline. *J Alzheimers Dis*. 2012; 30(Suppl 2): S147–s162. doi: 10.3233/JAD-2011-111028.

459 Schultz BG, Patten DK, Berlau DJ. The role of statins in both cognitive impairment and protection against dementia: a tale of two mechanisms. *Transl Neurodegener*. 2018 Feb 27; 7: 5. doi: 10.1186/s40035-018-0110-3.

460 Ma MM, Xu YY, Sun LH, et al. Statin-Associated Liver Dysfunction and Muscle Injury: Epidemiology, Mechanisms, and Management Strategies. *Int J Gen Med*. 2024 May 11; 17: 2055–2063. doi: 10.2147/IJGM.S460305.

461 Burri A, Maercker A, Krammer S, Simmen-Janevska K. Childhood trauma and PTSD symptoms increase the risk of cognitive impairment in a sample of former indentured child laborers in old age. *PLoS One*. 2013; 8(2): e57826. doi: 10.1371/journal.pone.0057826.

462 Seiler A, von Känel R, Slavich GM. The Psychobiology of Bereavement and Health: A Conceptual Review From the Perspective of Social Signal Transduction Theory of Depression. *Front Psychiatry*. 2020 Dec 3; 11: 565239. doi: 10.3389/fpsyt.2020.565239.

463 Brett BL, Gardner RC, Godbout J, Dams-O'Connor K, Keene CD. Traumatic Brain Injury and Risk of Neurodegenerative Disorder. *Biol Psychiatry*. 2022 Mar 1; 91(5): 498–507. doi: 10.1016/j.biopsych.2021.05.025.

464 Johnson VE, Stewart W. Traumatic brain injury: age at injury influences dementia risk after TBI. *Nat Rev Neurol*. 2015 Mar; 11(3): 128–130. doi: 10.1038/nrneurol.2014.241.

465 Franklin W, Krishnan B, Taglialatela G. Chronic synaptic insulin resistance after traumatic brain injury abolishes insulin protection from amyloid beta and tau oligomer-induced synaptic dysfunction. *Sci Rep*. 2019 Jun 3; 9(1): 8228. doi: 10.1038/s41598-019-44635-z.

466 Wright MJ, McArthur DL, Alger JR, et al. Early metabolic crisis-related brain atrophy and cognition in traumatic brain injury. *Brain Imaging Behav*. 2013 Sep; 7(3): 307–315. doi: 10.1007/s11682-013-9231-6.

467 Langer LK, Alavinia SM, Lawrence DW, et al. Prediction of risk of prolonged post-concussion symptoms: Derivation and validation of the TRICORDRR (Toronto Rehabilitation Institute Concussion Outcome Determination and Rehab Recommendations) score. *PLoS One*. 2021 Jul 8; 18(7): e1003652. doi: 10.1371/journal.pmed.1003652.

468 Goderez BI. Treatment of Traumatic Brain Injury With Hyperbaric Oxygen Therapy. *Psychiatric Times*. 2019 May 28; 36(5).

469 Gray SN. An Overview of the Use of Neurofeedback Biofeedback for the Treatment of Symptoms of Traumatic Brain Injury in Military and Civilian Populations. *Med Acupunct*. 2017 Aug 1; 29(4): 215–219. doi: 10.1089/acu.2017.

470 Cankaya S, Gunal M, Beker M, et al. The neuroprotective effect of Coconut Oil in mice with Traumatic Brain Injury. *Kahramanmaraş Sütçü İmam Üniversitesi Tıp Fakültesi Dergisi*. 2021. doi: 10.17517/ksutfd.853830.

471 Ibrahim KS, El-Sayed EM. Beneficial Effects of Coconut Oil in Treatment of Parkinson's Disease. *Neurophysiology*. 52: 169-175. doi: 10.1007/s11062-020-09866-1.

472 Masino SA, Kawamura M, Wasser CD, Pomeroy LT, Ruskin DN. Adenosine, ketogenic diet and epilepsy: the emerging therapeutic relationship between metabolism and brain activity. *Curr Neuropharmacol*. 2009 Sep; 7(3): 257–268. doi: 10.2174/157015909789152164.

473 Stein DG. Progesterone exerts neuroprotective effects after brain injury. *Brain Res Rev*. 2008 Mar; 57(2): 386–397. doi: 10.1016/j.brainresrev.2007.06.012.

474 Hamstra SI, Roy BD, Tiidus P, et al. Beyond its Psychiatric Use: The Benefits of Low-dose Lithium Supplementation. *Curr Neuropharmacol*. 2023; 21(4): 891–910. doi: 10.2174/1570159X20666220302151224.

475 Silver JM, McAllister TW, Yudofsky SC, eds. *Textbook of Traumatic Brain Injury, 3rd ed*. American Psychiatric Publishing; 2019.

476 Hadanny A, Abbott S, Suzin G, Bechor Y, Efrati S. Effect of hyperbaric oxygen therapy on chronic neurocognitive deficits of post-traumatic brain injury patients: retrospective analysis. *BMJ Open*. 2018 Sep 28; 8(9): e023387. doi: 10.1136/bmjopen-2018-023387.

477 Gray SN. An Overview of the Use of Neurofeedback Biofeedback for the Treatment of Symptoms of Traumatic Brain Injury in Military and Civilian Populations. *Med Acupunct*. 2017 Aug 1; 29(4): 215–219. doi: 10.1089/acu.2017.1220.

478 American Academy of Neurology. How Yoga Can Help People with Traumatic Brain Injury. February/March 2020.

479 Visit loveyourbrain.com for a TBI-specific yoga program.

480 Sullivan MB, Erb M, Schmalzl L, Moonaz S, Noggle Taylor J, Porges SW. Yoga therapy and polyvagal theory: The convergence of traditional wisdom and contemporary neuroscience for self-regulation and resilience. *Front Hum Neurosci*. 2018; 12(67). doi: 10.3389/fnhum.2018.00067.

481 Tani Y, Fujiwara T, Kondo K. Association Between Adverse Childhood Experiences and Dementia in Older Japanese Adults. *JAMA Net Open*. 2020 Feb 5; 3(2): e1920740. doi: 10.1001/jamanetworkopen.2019.20740.

482 Yehuda R, Daskalakis NP, Lehrner A, et al. Influences of maternal and paternal PTSD on epigenetic regulation of the glucocorticoid receptor gene in Holocaust survivor offspring. *Am J Psychiatry*. 2014 Aug; 171(8): 872–880. doi: 10.1176/appi.ajp.2014.13121571.

483 Bhattacharya S, Fontaine A, MacCallum PE, Drover J, Blundell J. Stress Across Generations: DNA Methylation as a Potential Mechanism Underlying Intergenerational Effects of Stress in Both Post-traumatic Stress Disorder and Pre-clinical Predator Stress Rodent Models. *Front Behav Neurosci*. 2019 May 28; 13: 113. doi: 10.3389/fnbeh.2019.00113.

484 Yaffe K, Vittinghoff E, Lindquist K, et al. Posttraumatic Stress Disorder and Risk of Dementia Among US Veterans. *Arch Gen Psychiatry*. 2010; 67(6): 608–613.

485 Anda RF, Felitti VJ, Bremner JD, et al. The enduring effects of abuse and related adverse experiences in childhood. A convergence of evidence from neurobiology and epidemiology. *Eur Arch Psychiatry Clin Neurosci*. 2006 Apr; 256(3): 174–186.

486 Burri A, Maercker A, Krammer S, Simmen-Janevska K. Childhood Trauma and PTSD Symptoms Increase the Risk of Cognitive Impairment in a Sample of Former Indentured Child Laborers in Old Age. *PLoS One*. 2013; 8(2): e57826.

487 Qureshi SU, Long ME, Bradshaw MR, et al. Does PTSD impair cognition beyond the effect of trauma? *J Neuropsychiatry Clin Neurosci*. 2011 Winter; 23(1): 16–28.

488 Gatchel JR, Rabin JS, Buckley RF, et al. Harvard Aging Brain Study. Longitudinal Association of Depression Symptoms With Cognition and Cortical Amyloid Among Community-Dwelling Older Adults. *JAMA Netw Open*. 2019 Aug 2; 2(8): e198964. doi: 10.1001/jamanetworkopen.2019.8964.

489 Hakim A. Perspectives on the complex links between depression and dementia. *Front Aging Neurosci*. 2022 Aug 24; 14:821866. doi: 10.3389/fnagi.2022.821866.

490 Banerjee S, High J, Stirling S, et al. Study of mirtazapine for agitated behaviours in dementia (SYMBAD): A randomised, double-blind, placebo-controlled trial. *Lancet Public Health*. 2021; 398(10310): 1487–1497. doi: 10.1016/S0140-6736(21)01210-1.

491 Wallensten J, Ljunggren G, Nager A, et al. Stress, depression, and risk of dementia – a cohort study in the total population between 18 and 65 years old in Region Stockholm. *Alzheimers Res Ther*. 2023 Oct 2; 15(1): 161. doi: 10.1186/s13195-023-01308-4.

492 Felitti VJ, Anda RF, Nordenberg D, et al. Relationship of childhood abuse and household dysfunction to many of the leading causes of death in adults. The Adverse Childhood Experiences (ACE) Study. *Am J Prev Med*. 1998 May; 14(4): 245–258. doi: 10.1016/s0749-3797(98)00017-8.

493 Danese A, J Lewis S. Psychoneuroimmunology of Early-Life Stress: The Hidden Wounds of Childhood Trauma? *Neuropsychopharmacology*. 2017 Jan; 42(1): 99–114. doi: 10.1038/npp.2016.198.

494 Puterman E, Gemmill A, Karasek D, et al. Lifespan adversity and later adulthood telomere length in the nationally representative US Health and Retirement Study. *Proc Natl Acad Sci USA*. 2016 Oct 18; 113(42): E6335–E6342. doi: 10.1073/pnas.1525602113.

495 Joseph J, Buss C, Knop A, et al. Greater maltreatment severity is associated with smaller brain volume with implication for intellectual ability in young children. *Neurobiol Stress*. 2023 Sep 23; 27: 100576. doi: 10.1016/j.ynstr.2023.100576.

496. Felitti VJ, Anda RF, Nordenberg D, et al. Relationship of childhood abuse and household dysfunction to many of the leading causes of death in adults. The Adverse Childhood Experiences (ACE) Study. *Am J Prev Med*. 1998 May; 14(4): 245–258. doi: 10.1016/s0749-3797(98)00017-8.

497. Davis S. A Closer Look at the Symptoms of Complex Post-Traumatic Stress Disorder. CPTSDfoundation.org. Published September 30, 2019. Accessed March 25, 2025. https://cptsdfoundation.org/2019/09/30/a-closer-look-at-the-symptoms-of-complex-post-traumatic-stress-disorder.

498. Rusk IL. Healing Trauma by Focusing on the Body. Ilenenaormirusk.com. Published March 5, 2020. Accessed March 25, 2025. https://sharpagain.org/healing-from-trauma-by-focusing-on-the-body.

499. Levine P. *In an Unspoken Voice: How the Body Releases Trauma and Restores Goodness.* North Atlantic Books; 2010.

500. van der Kolk BA. *The Body Keeps the Score: Brain, Mind, and Body in the Healing of Trauma.* Viking; 2014.

501. Grand D. *Brainspotting: The Revolutionary New Therapy for Rapid and Effective Change.* Sounds True; 2013.

502. Shapiro F. *Eye Movement Desensitization and Reprocessing (EMDR) Therapy, Third Edition: Basic Principles, Protocols, and Procedures.* Guilford Press; 2017.

503. Rusk IL. Trust Your Gut. Ilenenaormirusk.com. Published August 13, 2020. Accessed March 25, 2025. https://www.ilenenaomirusk.com/post/trust-your-gut-harnessing-the-power-of-interoception.

Index

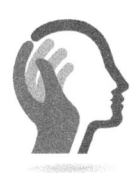

A

acetylcholine, 96
Acremonium, 157
acupuncture, for TBI, 188
AD. *See* Alzheimer's disease
addiction, 178
adenosine buildup, 64, 71
adenosine triphosphate (ATP), 177
ADHD (attention-deficit/hyperactivity disorder), 29, 60
adrenal glands, 95
adverse childhood experiences (ACEs), 181, 190, 192–193
aerobic exercise, 41–42, 46
AGEs (advanced glycation end products), 103
agricultural chemicals, 114–115
airborne pollutants, 106–108, 121–122
airway sleep disorders, 62–63, 68–69. *See also* sleep and breathing
alcohol, 28–29, 72
allergens, food, 37–38
aluminum, 137–138
Alzheimer, Alois, 201
Alzheimer's disease (AD), 11, 102–103
    See also brain health; cognitive function; dementia; memory loss
    advances in testing, 11
    aluminum exposure and, 137–138
    benzodiazepines and, 173, 175–176
    caffeine and, 24–25
    cholesterol and, 99–100, 101–102
    concussive trauma and, 182–183
    defined, 7
    diet and, 25–34
    dietary strategies for, 34–36
    EMF exposure, 108–111
    genes and epigenetics, 10–11
    heavy metal toxicity and, 130–131
    hormones and, 91–92
    inflammatory response, 147–148
    insulin and, 102–103
    ketones and, 185–186
    mental stimulation and, 51–54
    MIND diet, 22–23
    misdiagnosis of, 148
    neurosteroids and, 97–98
    oral hygiene and, 160
    pesticides and herbicides and, 114–115
    physical activities and, 41–48
    Porphyromonas gingivalis and, 160
    renewed hope for treatment, 201–202
    sleep quality and, 61–74
    sports injuries and, 189
    stress and, 77–78
    supplements, 36–38
    toxin-related, 115
    trans fats and, 116
    trauma and, 181–182
    Type 3 diabetes and, 103

amalgam fillings, 111, 133–134, 141–145
amyloid beta, 213
amyloid plaques, 31–32
antibiotics, gut flora and, 164
anticholinergics, 173–175
anti-inflammatories, 169
ApoE4 allele
    air pollution and, 107–108
    alcohol and, 28
    biomarkers, 149
    cardiovascular disease and, 10
    cholesterol management and, 102
    heavy metal toxicity and, 131–132
    inflammation and, 149
ApoE4 carriers, fasting and, 35
ApoE4 gene, DDT and, 30
Arestin (low-dose doxycycline), 162
arsenic, 138–139
arteries, hardening of, 61–62
artificial food ingredients, 29, 32–33, 112, 114, 123, 153
artificial light, sleep quality and, 72
aspartame, 112
aspergillus, 156, 157
atherosclerosis, 100, 133
ATP molecules, 185–186
attention-deficit/hyperactivity disorder (ADHD), 29
autoimmune disease, 94, 157, 168, 207
autonomic nervous system, 191

B

B vitamins, 37
BDNF (brain-derived neurotrophic factor), 19, 39
bedroom environment, sleep and, 73, 74
benzodiazepines, 173, 175–176
beryllium, 139
beta amyloid, 31–32, 61–62, 77–78
bifidobacterium breve M-16V, 120
bifidobacterium *infantis*, 119
biofeedback, for TBI, 188
black mold, 156, 157
blood cholesterol management, 101–102
blood lead levels (BLLs), 132
blood pressure, cognitive decline and, 31
blood sugar levels, 32, 33, 102–103
blood–brain barrier, 61
blunt force trauma, 182
body mass, 34–35
body-focused trauma recovery, 197–198
brain atrophy, 65–66
brain cholesterol metabolism, 177
brain-derived neurotrophic factor (BDNF), 19, 39
breathing problems, 62–63. *See also* sleep and breathing
Bredesen, Dale, 39, 206

C

cadmium, 139
caffeine, 24–25, 71
calories, 22, 32, 34–35
carbohydrates
    in alcohol, 28
    cognition and, 34–35
    fermentable, 163
    food sensitivities and, 150
    insulin and, 102
    Ketogenic diet, 35–36
    periodontal disease and, 161
    processed, 33–34
    refined, 31
cardio exercise, 46
cardiovascular health
    ApoE4 allele and, 10
    cholesterol and, 100
    heart-healthy diet, 22–23
    memory loss and, 9
    periodontal disease and, 159–160
    salt and cognitive decline, 31
    sugar substitutes and, 32–33
caregivers, 56, 79, 85
casein, 112
CDC (Centers for Disease Control and Prevention), 132, 154–155, 193
central nervous system
    air pollution and, 107
    anticholinergics and, 174
    electromagnetic frequency (EMF), 108–111
    inflammation and, 184
    microplastics and, 119

Omega 3s and, 186
VOCs and, 117
Cesarean births, 150
Chaetomium, 157
children. *See also* adverse childhood experiences (ACEs)
   ADHD and, 29
   EMF exposure and, 110
   emotional trauma and, 190, 191
   exposure to toxins, 108, 115–118
   food additives and, 29, 113
   HIIT training, 42–43
   lead toxicity and, 132
   Lyme disease and, 153–154
   mercury toxicity in, 133, 135
   mold exposure and, 156
   phthalates exposure and, 114
   sleep and breathing, 60–61, 67
   VOCs exposure, 117
chocolate, 29–30
cholesterol
   blood cholesterol management, 101–102
   HDL, 99–100, 177
   LDL, 99–100, 160
   lipids and, 99–100
   monitoring and management of, 100, 101–102
   prescription drugs and, 176–178
chromium, 139
chronic disease, 55–56, 110–111
chronic inflammation
   causes of, 147–149
   food sensitivities and, 151–152
   glycation and, 103
   heavy metals and, 139
   insulin and, 102–103
   memory loss and, 4
   sleep-disordered breathing and, 59–60
chronic stress
   ACEs and, 193
   brain function and, 76–77, 78
   inflammation and, 168
   PTSD and, 191–192
   trauma and, 181–182
circadian rhythm, 64, 65
Cladosporium, 156

Clean Fifteen, 30, 122–123
cleaning products toxicity, 116–117
coconut oil, 25, 185–186
cognitive function. *See also* Alzheimer's disease; dementia; memory loss
   air pollution and, 107–108
   cholesterol levels and, 99–100, 101–102, 176–178
   diet and foods, 22–23, 24–28, 30, 111–116
   dual-task training, 19
   environmental toxins and, 116–118
   improvement of, 52–53
   insulin and, 102–103
   lead levels and, 132
   low sodium and, 31
   nitrogen dioxide (NO2) and, 108, 117
   pesticides and herbicides and, 114–115
   prescription drugs and, 173–178
   rehabilitation, 51–52
   sleep and, 62
   stress and, 80–82
   studies related to, 17–19
   TBI and, 80–82, 183–184
   trauma and, 181–182, 195
cognitive reserve, 52–53
cognitive stimulation, 51–52
cognitive training, 19, 52
combat veterans, PTSD and, 195
complex post-traumatic stress disorder (C-PTSD), 193, 195
concussive injury, 182. *See also* traumatic brain injury
Consumer Confidence Report (drinking water), 120–121
CoQ10 (ubiquinone), 165–166, 177
corticosteroids, 77
cortisol, 76–80, 84, 181, 191
cosmetics, chemicals in, 118
COVID pandemic, 56–57
CPAP therapy, 62–63
C-reactive protein, 148, 159–160
creeping circadian rhythm, 65
CSE exercise (closed-skill environments), 41
curcumin, 169
cysteine, 112
cytokines, 77

D

daily sleep/wake cycle, 64
dance program study, 18–19
DASH-MIND diet, 22–23
deep sleep decline, 65
delayed stress, 79
dementia. *See also* Alzheimer's disease; cognitive function; memory loss
   air pollution and, 107–108
   airway sleep disorders and, 59–60, 67–68
   defined, 7
   depression and, 191–192
   electromagnetic frequency (EMF) and, 108–111
   glyphosate and, 115
   gum disease and, 160
   hormones and, 91–92
   inflammation and, 149
   insulin and, 102–103
   lipidology and, 100
   misdiagnosis of, 148
   populations at risk, 79
   risk factors for, 17–19
   social isolation and, 56
   stress levels and, 77–78
   TBI and, 191–192
   trans fats and, 116
   traumatic events and, 181–182
   veterans and, 191–192
demineralization, glyphosate and, 115
dental fillings, 111, 133–134, 136, 141–145
depression
   adverse childhood experiences (ACEs) and, 193
   EMF exposure and, 109–110
   emotional trauma and, 190–192
   food additives and, 112
   heavy metals toxicity and, 131
   inflammation and, 191–192
   Kirtan Kriya and, 85–87
   PTSD and, 191–192
   sleep fragmentation and, 66
   social interaction and, 55–56
   stress and, 76–77
   TBI and, 182–188
   yoga and, 44

detoxification
   breathing and sleep, 59–61
   daily regimen for, 125–126, 140–141
   EMFs and, 110
   exercise and, 40–41
   heavy metals and, 129–130, 131–133
   methylation cycle and, 106
   through the glymphatic system, 65
diabetes
   artificial sweeteners and, 32–33
   foods related to, 30–34
   insulin and, 102–103
   periodontal disease and, 159–160, 167
   Type 3, 103
diet and nutrition. *See also* nutrition and supplements
   additives, 29, 113
   alcohol, 28–29, 72
   artificial coloring, 113
   Clean Fifteen, 30
   DASH diet, 22
   Dirty Dozen, 30
   elimination diets, 151–152
   fasting, intermittent, 22, 34–35
   fermented foods, 120, 152–153
   fish consumption, 28, 135
   fish oil supplements, 37, 186
   flavanols, 29–30
   flavor enhancers, 113
   food additives, 112–113
   gluten sensitivity, 31
   healthy fats, 25–26
   heart-healthy diet, 22–23
   heavy metal toxicity, 141
   herbicides in food, 30, 114–115
   herbs and spices, 22, 26, 125–126, 166
   high glycemic foods, 33–34
   hydrogenated fats, 25, 116
   inflammation and, 37–38, 148–149, 168–169, 168t
   ketogenic diet, 22, 35–36
   ketones and, 185–186
   mercury found in foods, 135
   MIND diet, 22–23, 24t
   oral health and, 163–164, 165
   organic produce, 30

overeating, 62
processed foods, 21
protocol for brain health, 21-22
refined carbohydrates, 31, 33, 168, 179
SMASH fish, 28
standard American diet (SAD), 150-151
strategies and considerations, 28-37
sugar alcohols, 32-33
sugar consumption, 31-33
sugar substitutes, 32-33, 112
supplements, 36-37
toxic exposure and, 111-116, 122-123
toxins and, 125-126
trigger foods, 93
unhealthy fats, 34
whole grains, 30-31
Dietary Approaches to Stop Hypertension (DASH) diet, 22
dietary supplements, 36-37
digital screens, sleep quality and, 72
Dirty Dozen, 30, 122-123
drinking water supplies, 119, 120-121, 137-139
drug dependence, 178
dual-task training, 19
dysfunctional breathing patterns, 62-63

E

echinacea, 166
electromagnetic frequency (EMF), 108-111, 122
elimination diets, 151-152
EMDR (Eye Movement Desensitization and Reprocessing), 198
emotional dysregulation, 183-184
emotional trauma
    adverse childhood experiences (ACEs), 192-193
    body-focused trauma recovery, 197-198
    overview, 190
    physiological changes caused by, 191
    PTSD and, 191-192
    restorative yoga for, 198-199
    stress and, 80
    symptoms of, 193-196
    treatment for, 196
    The End of Alzheimer's Program (Bredesen), 39

endocrine disrupting chemicals (EDCs), 118
endodontic diseases, 163-164
Environmental Protection Agency (EPA), 106, 117, 120
environmental relative moldiness index (ERMI) test, 158
environmental toxins, 116-118, 156-158
Environmental Working Group Seafood Guide, 135
enzyme immunoassay (EIA) test, 155
epigenetic change, trauma and, 191
epilepsy, ketogenic diet and, 36
Epsom salts, 169
Epworth Sleepiness questionnaire, 69
erectile dysfunction, 96
essential oils, 162-163
estrogens, 95-98
excitotoxins, 112-113
executive function, 182-183, 188
exercise, 46-47, 71, 165, 186. *See also* physical activity
Eye Movement Desensitization and Reprocessing (EMDR), 198

F

fasting, intermittent, 22, 34-35
fermented foods, 120, 152-153
fetal development, 116
fibrillary tangles, 77-78
fight-or-flight response, 76-77, 197
Finnish Geriatric Intervention Study to Prevent Cognitive Impairment and Disability (FINGER), 17-18
fish consumption, 28, 135
fish oil supplements, 37, 186
flavanols, 29-30
flavor enhancers, 112-113
Flint, Michigan, lead levels, 132
folic acid, 166
food allergens, 37-38
Food and Drug Administration (FDA)
    changing priorities of, 106
    excitotoxins acceptable to, 113
    fish consumption advisory, 135
    trans fats and, 116
food consumption, sleep and, 72
food contamination, 29-30

food packaging, 114
food sensitivity, 22, 94, 150-153
foods. *See* diet and nutrition
forever chemicals, 120
formaldehyde, 117
functional medicine practitioners, 203-206
Functionalsource.com, 204

G

gasp reflex, 63
genetically modified organisms (GMOs), 21
glucose, 182-183, 185-186
glucose metabolism, 102-103
glutamate, 182
gluten sensitivity, 31
glycation system, 103
glycemic index (GI), 33-34
glycemic load (GL), 33-34
glymphatic system, 61, 64, 65
glyphosate weed killer, 115
GMOs (genetically modified organisms), 21
good bacteria, 152-153
grain consumption, 30-31
grape seed extract (GSE), 166
gum disease, 160
gut health
 antibiotics and, 164
 bifidobacteria in, 120
 brain health and, 111
 elimination diet and, 37-38
 fermented foods and, 120
 glyphosate and, 115
 grains and, 31
 gut microbiome, 150-152
 gut microbiota dysbiosis, 120
 inflammatory foods and, 95
 leaky gut, 94, 150
gut-brain axis, 27-28

H

hardening of arteries, 61-62
Hashimoto's Thyroiditis, 93-94
HbA1c test, 149
HDL cholesterol, 99-100, 177
head trauma. *See* traumatic brain injury (TBI)
health effects roster of type-specific formers of mycotoxins and inflammagens (HERTSMI) test, 158
healthcare professionals, 203-206
healthy eating habits, 167
healthy fats, 25-26
healthy lifestyle, 17-19
heart health, 99-100. *See also* cardiovascular health
heart-healthy diet, 22-23
heat, to reduce inflammation, 169
heavy metal (HM) toxicity
 accumulation in the body, 131-132
 aluminum, 137-138
 arsenic, 138-139
 in chocolate bars, 29-30
 dangers of, 130-131
 foods, supplements, and therapies, 141
 heavy metals defined, 130
 lead, 132
 mercury, 132-137
 others, 139
 overview, 129-130
 ridding the body of, 140-145
 signs and symptoms, 131-132, 136-137
 testing for, 139-140
herbicide toxicity, 30, 114-115
herbs, to treat inflammation, 169
herbs and spices, 22, 26, 125-126, 166, 169
HERTSMI mold test, 158
high glycemic foods, 33-34
high-intensity interval training (HIIT), 42-43, 46
high-sensitivity C-reactive protein (hs-CRP) test, 148, 159-160
hippocampal atrophy, 78
holistic practitioners, 203-206
home environment toxins, 116-118, 123-124, 156-158
homocysteine levels, 149
hormones
 brain health and, 97-99
 cholesterol, 101-102
 hunger hormones, 62
 inflammation and, 97-98
 insulin, 102-103
 overview, 91-92

satiety hormones, 62
sex hormones, 95-97
stress hormones, 191
hydration, 22, 26-27
hydrogenated fats, 25, 116
hyperactivity, 29
hyperbaric oxygen, for TBI, 187-188
hypopenea, 63
hypothyroidism, 92-93, 93t
hypoxia, 60-61, 68-69

I

IgE (immunoglobulin E) test, 151
IgG (immunoglobulin G) blood test, 151
immune response, 149
immune system, 115, 150, 165-167, 193
immune-excitotoxicity, mercury and, 133
immunofluorescent assay (IFA) test, 155
immunoglobulin tests, 37-38
infection, thyroid function and, 95
inflammation
    anti-inflammatories, 169
    asymptomatic, 149
    dementia and, 149
    depression and, 191-192
    diet-related, 22, 37-38
    exercise and, 167
    food consumption and, 30
    glycation and, 103
    heat and ice to reduce, 169
    herbs to treat, 169
    hormones and, 97-98
    post-concussion syndrome and, 183-185
    stress and, 79, 80
inflammation and infections
    detecting, 148-149
    food sensitivities, 150-153
    Lyme disease, 153-155
    mold exposure, 156-158
    oral infections, 159-167
    overview, 147-148
    systemic, 168-169, 168t
    urinary tract infections, 167
inflammatory foods, 95
innate immune system, 115
insect repellent, 155

insomnia, 66. *See also* sleep and breathing
insulin, concussive trauma and, 182-183
insulin hormones, 102-103
insulin resistance, 22, 25, 31-32
integrative healthcare practitioners, 203-206
intermittent fasting, 22, 34-35
intermittent nocturnal oxygen deprivation, 63

J

Johns Hopkins University study, 147-148

K

Kaiser Permanents ACEs study, 193
ketogenic diet, 22, 35-36
ketones, 25, 185-186
Kirtan Kriya (KK) meditation, 85-87

L

The Lancet
    air pollution study, 107
LDL cholesterol, 99, 100, 160
lead, 132
leaky gut, 94, 150-151
libido, 97
lifestyle practices
    mental stimulation, 51-54
    nutrition and supplements, 21-38
    overview, 17-19
    physical activity, 39-50
    risk factors, 17-19
    sleep and breathing, 59-74
    social interaction, 55-57
lipids, cholesterol and, 99-100
Loma Linda University nutritional supplements study, 165
Lyme disease, 153-155

M

MCTs (medium-chain triglycerides), 25, 185-186
meditation, 43-44, 47, 84-87
Mediterranean Intervention for Neurodegenerative Delay (MIND) diet, 22-23, *24t*
medium-chain triglycerides (MCTs), 25, 34

melatonin, 73
memory consolidation, 64–65
memory loss. *See also* Alzheimer's disease; cognitive function; dementia
    cortisol and, 77–78
    EMF exposure and, 109
    Lyme disease and, 154
    meditation and, 84, 85
    mold exposure and, 156, 157
    populations at risk, 79
    potential for reversal, 8, 16
    risk factors, 8–9
    stress and, 77–78
    TBI and, 182
    vitamin E and, 36
memory recall, 61
menopause, 96, 97–98
men's health, 95-98
mental stimulation, 51–54
mercury, 132–137, 139–140
mercury amalgam removal, 141–145
messaging molecules, 91
metabolic processes, 91
methylation cycle, 106
microbial colonic community composition, 119
microplastics, 118–119
MIND-DASH diet, 22–23
mindfulness and meditation, 84–85
mold exposure and testing, 156–158
monosodium glutamate (MSG), 112–113
monounsaturated fats, 25, 27
Monsanto, glyphosate and, 115
mood issues, TBI and, 183
mood medications, 178
mouth breathing, 60, 63
MSG (monosodium glutamate), 112–113
MTHFR (methylenetetrahydrofolate reductase), 106
multidomain lifestyle intervention, 17–18
mycotoxins, 156

N

nanoplastics, 118–119
naps, sleep quality and, 71
National Institutes of Health (NIH), 120

negative thinking, stress and, 79
neuro-cognitive risk, 68–69
neurofeedback (NF), for TBI, 188
neurological diseases, 107, 112, 131, 182
neurological pathologies, mercury and, 133–134
neurosteroids, 97–98
neurotoxicity process, 182
nickel, 139
nitrogen dioxide (NO2), 108, 117
nonnutritive sweeteners (NNS), 32–33
non-rapid eye movement (NREM), 64
nonstick pans, 117–118
NREM sleep, 61
nutraceuticals, for TBI, 187
nutrition and supplements. *See also* diet and nutrition
    brain-healthy foods, 24–28
    dietary strategies and considerations, 28–37
    diet-related inflammation, 37–38
    food allergies, 37–38
    foods to monitor, minimize, or eliminate, 28–34
    gut health, 37–38
    melatonin, 73
    MIND diet, 22–23, 24t
    overview, 21–22
    phenylalanine (in aspartame), 112
    recommended dietary protocol, 21–22
    thyroid function and, 95

O

obstructive sleep apnea (OSA), 62–63
Ohio University stress study, 79
olive oil, 27
Omega 3 fatty acids, 37, 186
oral appliance therapy, 62–63
oral health, 159–167, 160
organic produce, benefits of, 30
OSE exercise (open-skill environments), 41
oxidative stress, 31, 62
oxygen deprivation, 59–60, 61–62

P

pain medication, 178

parasympathetic state, stress and, 76
penicillium, 157
periodontal diseases, 159-163
peroxide gel treatment, 162
personal care products, 118, 124
pesticides, 30, 114-115
PFAS chemicals, 117-118, 120
phenylalanine (in aspartame), 112
phenylketonuria (PKU), 112
phthalates, 114
physical activity
    aerobic exercise, 40-42, 46
    benefits of, 48-49
    guidelines for starting, 45, 48
    HIIT training, 42-43, 46
    OSE vs. CSE exercise, 41
    overview, 39
    Qigong, 44-45, 47
    resistance training, 43, 46
    self-assessment and planning, 47-48
    stability/flexibility/mind-body, 43, 46
    strength training, 43, 46
    Tai Chi, 44-45, 47
    thyroid function and, 95
    yoga and Pilates, 43-44, 47
physical stress, 80
physical trauma. See traumatic brain injury (TBI)
physiological stress response, 195-196
Pilates, 43-44, 47
placebo effect, sleep quality and, 73
plaque, periodontal disease and, 161-162
plastics, 118-120, 124-125
polypropylene, 119
polyunsaturated fats, 25-26
Porphyromonas gingivalis, 160
post-concussion syndrome, 183-184
post-traumatic stress disorder (PTSD), 191-192
power plant pollutants, 134-135
prebiotics and probiotics, 27-28, 152-153
prenatal mercury exposure, 133
prescription drugs
    cognitive function and, 173-178
    new medications, 172-173
    overview, 171-172
    reducing dosage and ceasing, 178-179
    sleep aids, 73
    for TBI, 187
proanthocyanidins, 166-167
probiotics, 119, 152-153
processed foods, 21, 33
progesterone, 95-97, 97-98
prolonged stress
    cortisol, 77-78
    identification of stressors, 78-82
    impact on the brain, 76-77
    managing, 82-87
    overview, 75
psychotherapy, 79-80
PTSD (post-traumatic stress disorder), 191-192

Q
Qigong, 44-45, 47, 190
quantitative EEG (qEEG), 188

R
rapid eye movement (REM), 64
reduced dosing, 178-179
refined carbohydrates, 31, 33, 161, 168, 179
reptilian brain, stress and, 77
resistance training, 19, 46
rest, thyroid function and, 95
rest and gentle exercise, TBI and, 186
restorative yoga, 188, 198-199
root canal treatments, 163
Roundup weed killer, 115

S
salt consumption, 31
satiety hormones, 62
saturated fats, 34, 101
Schumann Resonance, 108-109
secondary sleep effects, 61-62
sedation, sleep aids and, 73
sensory disturbances, 183-184
sex hormones, 95-98
silver dental fillings, 133, 134, 136, 141-145
singing exercise, 85
sleep and breathing
    basics of sleep, 63-65

breathing and airway problems, 62-63
dementia and, 59-60
improving, 66-69, 69-70
overview, 59
problems with aging, 65-66
reduced oxygen levels and, 60-61
secondary sleep effects, 61-62
sleep hygiene, 70-74
sleep quality, 61, 67-68
snoring, 63
STOP-Bang sleep test, 69
TBI and, 183
testing, 69-70
sleep/wake cycle, 64
SMASH fish, 28
social isolation, 55-57
sodium caseinate, 112
sodium intake, 31
Somatic Experiencing (SE), 197-198
sports injuries, AD and, 189
spouse caregivers, 56
stachybotrys atra (black mold), 156
standard American diet (SAD), 150-151
statins, 101-102, 166, 173, 176-178
stool analysis, 152
STOP-Bang sleep test, 69
strength training, 46
stress
　delayed, 79
　depression and, 76-77
　inflammation and, 79, 80, 147
　management of, 82-84
　negative thinking and, 79
　parasympathetic state and, 76
　physiological response to, 195-196
　predispositions toward, 79
　reptilian brain and, 77
　signs and symptoms of, 80-82
　sources of, 78-79
　technology and, 80
　thyroid function and, 95
stress hormones, trauma and, 191
stress response, 197-198
sugar
　added, 32
　alcohols, 32-33

consumption, 31-33
substitutes, 32-33, 112
suicide, 193
sunlight, circadian rhythm and, 72
supplements. *See also* diet and nutrition
　benefits of, 185
　cognitive health and, 172
　to consider, 186
　CoQ10, 166, 177
　dietary, 36-37, 165-166
　heavy metals and, 141
　Omega 3, 186
　possible interactions, 173
　TBI and, 186
support-seeking behavior, 197
survival instincts, 197-198
sympathetic nervous system, 76
synthetic chemicals, 116-117
systemic inflammation
　detecting, 148-149
　Lyme disease and, 153-154
　periodontal disease and, 161-162
　secondary sleep effects and, 62
　treatment of, 168-169
　UTIs and, 168

T

T3 and T4 hormones, 4, 92
Tai Chi, 44-45, 47, 190
talk therapy, 196
tau proteins, 61, 77
TBI. *See* traumatic brain injury (TBI)
technology, stress and, 80
Teflon coating, 117-118
testosterone, 95-98
Tetrahydrocannabinol (THC), 73
threat defense systems, 197
thyroid, brain function and, 92-95
tick bites, 154-155
time-restricted feeding, 22, 34-35
toxic body burden, 95, 105, 125, 131
Toxic Substances Control Act (1976), 118
toxins. *See also* heavy metal (HM) toxicity
　in the air, 106-108, 121-122
　Alzheimer's disease and, 115
　broad spectrum testing for, 126

electromagnetic frequencies, 108–111, 122
in food, 30, 111–116, 122–123
home and work environments, 116–121, 123–124
indoor environment, 116–118, 123–124
mold, 158
overview, 105–106
in personal care products, 124
in plastics, 124–125
preventing exposure to, 121–125
sources and effects of exposure, 106–121
testing and treatment for, 125–126
in water, 125
traditional healthcare, 203–206
trans fats, 25, 34, 116
transgender and non-binary individuals (TNB), 79
trauma
body-focused recovery, 197
emotional trauma, 190–199
overview, 181–182
stored trauma, 198
traumatic brain injury (TBI), 182–190
unresolved, 195
trauma memories, 191
traumatic brain injury (TBI)
general symptoms, 183
ketones, 185–186
long-term effects, 183–184
Omega 3 supplements, 186
other supplements, 186
other treatment options, 187–188
overview, 182–183
preventing, 188–190
rest and gentle exercise, 186
treatment, 184–185
veterans and, 191–192
traumatic energy, 196
trigger foods, 93
turmeric, 169
Type 2 diabetes, 30
Type 3 diabetes, 103

U

UARS (upper airway resistance syndrome), 63
unhealthy fats, 34

University of Central Lancashire (UCLan) oral hygiene study, 160
University of Florida periodontal disease study, 160
University of Toronto air pollution study, 107
unresolved traumas, 195
unsaturated fats, 25–26
upper airway resistance syndrome (UARS), 63
urinary tract infections (UTI), 167
urine challenge text, 139–140
U.S. Surgeon General periodontal diseases study, 160

V

vaccines, 135
vaginal births, 150
vascular health, statins and, 176–178
veterans, PTSD and, 191–192
vitamins, 36–37, 149, 165–166, 186
volatile organic compounds (VOCs), 117

W

water contaminants, 120–121, 125
water filter technologies, 121
weight management, 101
weight training, 97
well water testing, 120–121
wellness coaches, 205
Western immunoblot test, 155
white blood cell count (WBC), 149
white matter damage, 147–148
whole grains, 30–31
women's health, 95–98
Women's Health Initiative Memory Study (WHIMS), 107–108
work environment toxins, 116–118, 123–124
World Health Organization (WHO), 39, 137–138

Y

yoga, 43–44, 47, 188, 190, 198–199

Z

zero blockage, 63

Thank you for reading this book;
please leave a review online at your preferred retail site.
Your review will help others find this book.

Visit sharpagain.org to:

- Download the *Sharp Again Roadmap to a Sharper Mind* and access other resources
- Register to participate in upcoming programs
- Donate to support and expand our work

Follow us on social media:

@SharpAgainNaturally

@SharpAgain

@SharpAgain6872